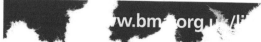

The Other Side
of Medicine

D1585736

To all my registrars and to my friends on the
RCGP Panel of Examiners, past and present

The Other Side of Medicine

Peter Tate

Retired Convenor,
MRCGP Examination

Radcliffe Publishing
Oxford • Seattle

Radcliffe Publishing Ltd
18 Marcham Road
Abingdon
Oxon OX14 1AA
United Kingdom

www.radcliffe-oxford.com
Electronic catalogue and worldwide online ordering facility.

British Library Cataloguing in Publication Data

A catalogue record for this book is available from the British Library.

ISBN-10: 1 84619 154 8
ISBN-13: 978 1 84619 154 1

Typeset by Anne Joshua & Associates, Oxford
Printed and bound by TJ International Ltd, Padstow, Cornwall

Contents

Preface

This book is a collection of articles and short stories covering a medical career. The bulk of the articles were published in *Education for Primary Care* between 2001 and 2006 under the heading 'Tate on Training.' Some of the essays are iconoclastic, the theme of good communication in medicine runs throughout, and other themes are quality in doctors and the assessment of that quality. However, I hope that the main strand of the book is humanity in medicine and my attempts at understanding what that is.

Peter Tate
Corfe Castle
August 2006
spudtate@supanet.com

About the author

Peter Tate qualified at the University of Newcastle in 1968. After spells as a P&O surgeon and as a trainee in Kentish Town, he worked as a GP in Abingdon for 30 years. He was a trainer from 1976 until 2003, and was also a course organiser in Oxford for eight years. He was an MRCGP examiner from 1981, and was responsible for the introduction of the video module in 1996. He retired as Convenor of the Panel of Examiners in March 2006. He was a co-author of *The Consultation* and *The New Consultation* (both published by Oxford University Press), and has lectured widely on communication issues. He is now semi-retired and lives in Corfe Castle.

Chapter 1

Does thinking make us stupid?

Cleverer people than I have mused on the evolutionary merits of intelligence. We have found no fossil trilobites with big brains, and they were around for aeons of geological time. Then the wonderfully big dinosaurs ate, fought and farted around (literally) for a huge time span without ever finding the need to develop mobile phones. So why in the last few seconds of geological time have we evolved intelligence?

Looked at dispassionately, intelligence has not been an unmitigated success. We can destroy ourselves on a scale undreamed of in the animal kingdom and, with our capacity to meddle on a large scale, we can now destabilise our planet even quicker than the vagaries of the cosmic forces that surround us. Human scientific progress is now happening on a scale so fast that makes no sense when compared to the relatively slow pace of evolution, even in human history. After all, since 'intelligence', progress is certainly not relentless. Those wonderful and esoteric Egyptians came from nowhere to instant technological wizardry, the Great Pyramid is still literally unbelievable, the second impressive but not as good and in no time they couldn't build them at all. They could still mould King Tut's awe-inspiring funerary mask 1000 years later, but they carried on going backwards slowly for another 1000 years till Cleopatra finished it off for good.

Ah, I hear you say, but what has all this to do with general practice? Well, my thesis relates to the dominance of intellectualism over instinct. The real problem is that we are not clever enough; our much vaunted intelligence is pretty superficial and to understand things at all we have to reduce complexities to simple building blocks, thus distorting the true nature of the phenomenon. The number of blocks gets nowhere near the mystery of the Great Pyramid; an equation cannot describe the beauty or the mind-numbing infiniteness of a Mandelbrot fractal. A Manchester rating scale cannot do justice to the subtleties of doctor–patient interactions, and a deep understanding of the Krebs cycle doesn't help most doctors to cure anyone. On top of this, we become ridiculously possessive and overbearing with the bits of knowledge we have gleaned. Take the health professions. Cholesterol is bad for you as is too much fat, smoking is anathema and obesity is a dangerous state. All such statements have some truth in them but take no account of values, human instinct or experience, and the real truth is much more complex, multivariate and capable of being viewed from many perspectives. Health messages become reduced to little more than slogans and the complex instinctive nature of human decision making is unacknowledged.

We have evolved to make decisions about situations and our fellows almost instantly, we are often attracted to another across a crowded room, sometimes we dislike on sight. We know from personal experience that our original impressions are mostly, but not always, confirmed. Human conversation is based on previous experience, unconscious observations, pheromones, feelings and hunches, but most of our teaching isn't. We are a funny bunch, opinionated, aggressive and irrational but forever vaunting our intelligence.

You may not have guessed it but the underlying theme of this piece is communication and how we learn it and teach it. We all learn how to communicate from a very early age, and most of us are not taught in the conventional sense. When our teachers do attack us with subjunctives, gerunds, past participles, split infinitives and tell us we can't boldly go, some of us are instinctively irritated, some of us make it a lifetime study and most just put such grammatical pontifications to the back of our mind to be remembered in exams and interviews but not important in our daily existence.

Now the thing is we are creatures with only a modicum of intelligence, but we do carry with us a barrel load of attitudes. What is an attitude? The OED says it is a *considered* and permanent disposition or reaction to a person or thing. I might quibble with considered as many attitudes I have are not considered, they just are, visceral, instinctive and sometimes clearly tribal. Some I am not proud of so I won't tell you what they are and I spend a lot of my life hiding some of these attitudes lest I end up with few friends . . . are you any different? Alan Bennett's wonderful *Talking Heads* series allows single human beings to display their naked attitudes for all to hear and makes for riveting, if depressing, entertainment; most human prejudices are attitudes too. Attitudes are only very loosely related to intelligence, they tend to come from the mid-brain, not the cortex; they are based on survival instincts and emotional feedback loops that are hard to dissect and often not amenable to logical understanding.

The point I wish to make about attitudes is that they govern our behaviour. Your heart may sink at this juncture and you may stop reading because this point is so obvious . . . all that for this! But, if you bear with me, I would just like to point out that most conventional educational theory implies, in some cases even states, that knowledge governs behaviour. The health educators are driven unceasingly (and fruitlessly) by this belief. I am not saying that knowledge does not change behaviour, but it only works when what is learned changes an attitude about, say, a procedure, a screening opportunity, or a loosely held attitude, say, for or against the legalisation of cannabis. This, of course, makes the point that not all attitudes are equal; some are much more entrenched than others and much less amenable to the voice of sweet reason. Here again I must disagree with the OED's use of the word *permanent*; attitudes do change, but usually slowly. Now, if we doctors concentrated on finding out the attitudes of our patients to the slings and arrows of outrageous medicine, we might be more effective in steering our patients to doing what is currently thought to be good for them. Of course, the same applies to us, we have attitudes too. When ours clash with those of our patients we can only rely on 'professionalism' to help us through it, followed by a strong cup of coffee and a gripe to our partners. Trying to find out what our patients' attitudes are implies that we are minded to do so, in other words we have an attitude to an attitude.

People's attitudes are not necessarily what they say they are. This again is not a revelation but an uneasy truth about a common lie. In the MRCGP oral examination, for many years, examiners were taught not just to expose the attitudes of the candidate, for or against termination, for example, but to seek for the justification of that attitude. The argument being that you can't really mark attitudes out of ten, but you can have a stab at rank ordering the justifications. This is not easy and one person's justification is another's bigotry. Justifications tend of course to be post hoc cortical intellectualisations of inherently mid-brain feelings. In the oral examination all candidates, without exception, claimed they believed in and practised the patient-centred method, and most could describe several consulting models and the concepts behind them to the satisfaction of the examiners. Then along came the video examination and only 10% could demonstrate actually doing it in the consultations they had selected to demonstrate just that. Here there is a breakdown in the theory; the stated attitudes do not lead to the stated behaviour, so the attitude must not be the real one, and candidates are fibbing. Why? This is one of the big questions for GP trainers and educators.

Practising patient-centred medicine is in fact pretty easy if you want to do it; you just have to listen, be curious and participate in a dialogue, not a monologue, but you do have to want to do it. Communication courses have, for years, used models of educational behaviour: tasks, strategies and skills abound. There have been many programmes full of skilful simulated patients, hours of dissecting videotapes, clever skill training workshops, and having witnessed 25 years of this sort of educational input personally as a trainer since 1976 and as an 'educator' contributing more than my fair share of tasks, performance criteria, etc., agonisingly slow changes in actual doctor behaviour. Again, why? The simple answer is that the majority of the profession still don't rate patient-centred, evidence-based, shared decision making as worth the time and emotional effort to them and, if they feel like that, all the knowledgeable clever teaching in the world is going to make no or, at most, very little difference.

Actually, the majority of humans, as I have previously intimated, don't need much teaching in communication. Many young registrars of my personal experience have become really 'good' communicators in the sense of involving their patients almost overnight, following a real attitude change brought on by an overbearing trainer or a realisation of the annoying consequences of failing the MRCGP video module. Of course, they can then improve, practise the skills till they become automatic and instinctive again, but the first and fundamental step is the change in attitude. If we think about our attitudes, then our intelligence might be useful. Get the attitude right by thinking, then let instinct, experience and evolution take over and the results are almost magical. John Lennon was wrong, all you need is attitude, but it has to be the right one, and there is the rub.

Chapter 2

What really matters?

We live in troubled times and this question is too broad for an easy answer. Dear old Maslow, the famous American humanistic psychologist, devised a six-level hierarchy of motives that, according to his theory, determine human behaviour. He ranked human needs as follows:

1 physiological
2 security and safety
3 love and feelings of belonging
4 competence, prestige, and esteem
5 self-fulfilment
6 curiosity and the need to understand.

His argument was that you start with need 1 and, if you are lucky, you progress to needs 5 and 6, which he unhelpfully labelled 'self-actualisation'. Currently, most western GPs, and those who aspire to be one, are lucky. If, however, you see this list as an allegory of forever climbing onwards and upwards, like climbing a skyscraper for example, then the shakiness of the structure is only too obvious since the events of 11 September 2001. We have to live for the good tomorrow and continue to self-actualise as much as we can, so how can we help our registrars on this crucial journey? Ed Peile, a GP near Aylesbury, and two colleagues have published a paper in a rival journal that set me thinking, surely the main purpose of journals.[1] The paper's title asks the important question: The year in a training practice: what has lasting value?

This is a personal column, so I considered my own story to see what had lasting value for me. I am able to look back with a reasonable depth of perspective because I was a registrar, trainee then, 30 years ago. A few personal details to set the scene: my dad was a single-handed GP, who had only my mother as help, as he consulted from a damp basement surgery in South Shields. He liked people, hated the NHS because of, as he perceived it, the Stalinistic second-class patronising nature of the whole organisation. He died, in harness, of myasthenia gravis aged 58. My experience of general practice was thus a cautionary one. When I qualified in 1968 I had no idea what I wished to do in medicine. Father was still working then and, though I loved him dearly, working with him in those conditions was not an attractive option. A bit of Maslow's needs 1 and 2 was missing. So I did what many young doctors have done. I dotted around, trying a bit of this and that to see if anything appealed to me as a life-long calling. I moved down to London, The Royal Northern Hospital Holloway Road to be precise, and found that Sunderland General was better than I had thought. I went away to sea as a ship's surgeon and was lucky enough to be promoted to senior surgeon on a big white P&O liner. The medicine was terrific, the responsibility awesome, the social life unbelievable, and the career prospects nil. A ship's surgeon is an old-fashioned GP; the job description is that you do everything that needs doing, with the help of your team. For the first time I began to think that I really wanted to be a GP. I got off the ship in 1972 and moved into a flat in Southampton Row W1, owned by my future wife. Training was not compulsory then and I toyed with going straight into practice; there were a couple of tempting offers, but a little inner voice told me that I was nowhere near the finished article and that I needed more help. I applied for a traineeship in Kentish Town and, against the odds, got it; to this day I can't get over how lucky I was. Curiously, I wrote to my trainer at the end of the year, this was to thank him and tell him what I had learned. I was his first registrar so I wished to be helpful. I still have a copy of this letter and my toes curl with embarrassment when re-reading it, but it does remind me of my short-term perspective.

So back to Ed Peile's question. What had lasting value?

Number one, without a shadow of a doubt, was the enthusiasm for general practice demonstrated by all in my training practice. This enthusiasm osmosed into my being over the year, and has remained there ever since. Looking back, I can dissect out bits of specific enthusiasms that were demonstrated to me. My trainer was currently sitting the MRCP examination, having gone into practice straight from pre-reg as you could in those days. To do this required an enormous amount of extra work, not just book reading, but ward rounds, etc. There was no obvious professional gain attached to this qualification for him at that time; it was a matter of pride and an external proof that Lord Moran was wrong about GPs just being those who were not good enough to climb the hospital ladder. I suppose the modern equivalent is the MSc or similar. The practice had two trainers, so I had the luxury of alternating tutorials, giving different experiences and different perspectives. I quickly discovered that my other trainer was very special too – a thinker, painter, polymath and an enthusiast for the College of General Practitioners. This was different for me; my father disliked the RCGP, certain that it was populated by self-seeking pompous people with inferiority complexes. This was a widely held view then, and is still current in some quarters. I learned then, and know now, that in that belief father was wrong. Before my first tutorial with trainer two, the trainer gave me a brand new book called *The Future General Practitioner: learning and teaching.*[2] He asked me to read chapters 2 and 3 on the consultation and then we would talk about it. He modestly asked for my opinion as he was the main author and worried that it might be difficult to follow. It was; I tried to do as he asked and, slowly, a creeping terror enveloped me – I hardly understood any of it. I read it again and again hoping for the light to dawn, but it didn't. At this stage of my life I was a sybarite, practical and un- but not anti-intellectual. This was clever stuff and I was not ready to understand it, but I was annoyed at myself for being so thick. This realisation that thinking was going to be a necessary prerequisite of good general practice was a much-needed jolt which has proved of lasting value. With the example set by both trainers, I started working too, and sat the still fairly new MRCGP examination at the end of the year. Something I had not even thought about on starting.

The same trainer introduced me to Balint; he was a member of the original group, and, although I have not become a true disciple myself, the insights about the drug doctor and the role of emotions in consulting were revelatory and permanent. Looking back, these experiences that related to thinking about consulting metaphorically took a lot of the stones from the ground and so, when I met David Pendleton some five years later, the seeds he sowed in my mind germinated because of my training practice experience.

I am lucky that my life is full of heroes. Henry Miller, the wonderful neurologist and dean of my medical school, was my first, and the aforementioned David P has the uneasy role of hero and friend, but my two trainers top my current lengthy list. This is not the same as role modelling; it is recognising special people who have enthused me in one way or another and so changed my life. This is not to say that all trainers must be heroes, but they should all be enthusiasts.

Ed Peile's paper dissects out helpful and unhelpful learning and teaching behaviours but, at a distance of 30 years, I can't remember much of the specifics, except for an overwhelming feeling of being accepted, listened to, and having my opinions valued. Ed would call that learner-centred teaching, and I have always tried to follow that example with my own registrars.

Re-reading my letter to my trainer, there were three areas I delineated that had most improved my ability to help people.

1 Listening properly to what patients say.
2 The skill of using time, both diagnostically and over a series of consultations, to understand people better.
3 Good note-keeping, described as the root from which all else grows. I can hear my partners' hollow laughter now.

I wonder what you have found of lasting value?

References

1   Peile EB, Easton GP and Johnson N (2001) The year in a training practice: what has lasting value? Grounded theoretical categories and dimensions from a pilot study. *Medical Teacher.* **23**(2): 205–11.
2   Horder J, Byrne P, Freeling P, Harris C, Irvine D and Marinker M (1972) *The Future General Practitioner: learning and teaching.* RCGP Publications: London.

Chapter 3

Assessment: is it good or bad for training?

When I first became a trainer in 1976 I was not very good. Not because I didn't know much educational theory, which I didn't, but mainly because I was not clear enough about what I did know that might be useful to my marginally more insecure registrar. I tried to read myself out of trouble, and fell upon an RCGP occasional paper by Denis Pereira-Grey (now Sir). This contained the famous triangular trilogy of Aims–Methods–Assessments. Defining the aims of vocational training or, more explicitly, the educational needs of GPs, as had been started by *The Future General Practitioner: learning and teaching*, the 1972 RCGP publication, would obviously lead to clear teaching methods that could then be properly assessed. As we all know, it has not turned out to be that easy. The first and major problem was getting trainers to agree on the important aims. This debate rumbled on and I became a course organiser in Oxford in 1978. After some years, the Thames Valley course organiser group, led by the dynamic John Hasler, tried to define these aims more clearly and produced another occasional paper called 'Priority objectives for general practice'. This was fundamentally a clarification and expansion of the *Future GP*, an attempted syllabus for the profession. Meanwhile, the Leeuwenhorst European working party had also expanded the *Future GP*, making 21 statements divided into knowledge, skills and attitudes, forming a job description of general practice. Lots of trainer assessment methodologies appeared too, the most lasting being the complex Manchester rating scales.

Training methods were, and remain, haphazard. These are still founded mainly in the apprenticeship tutorial model, relying heavily on random case analysis and really covering areas that the trainer and registrar feel comfortable about. Evidence accumulated over many years from the MRCGP examination, and studies from Glasgow, suggest that many, possibly most, trainers are not very good at assessing their own registrar's ability in some areas, especially their knowledge base and communication skills. So the hard, somewhat unpalatable, truth is that for most registrars the aims of the training year are relatively unclear, except to finish it with a valid certificate and perhaps the MRCGP qualification. The teaching methods will vary wildly from practice to practice, and even more so from region to region, and the amount of useful, valid and reliable formative assessments will in many cases be minimal.

As the nature of the job keeps changing, it is right and proper that various bodies continue to redefine what the discipline of general practice actually is and what its main constituents are. The currently constituted European Society of General Practice and WONCA Europe are doing it at present. But there has been a subtle change; aims have been replaced by basic principles leading to 'central characteristics', the performance of which can be defined by listing the core competencies. One such basic principle is seen as 'patient-centred care'. Now this is close to my heart and, other than learning the basic principles of medicine itself, is to me the most necessary characteristic that a GP can possess. It also seems to me that, in the finite time available to train the future GPs, this should be priority number one. There are, of course, at least a couple of snags. Firstly, not everyone agrees that this should be so; secondly, there are many definitions of patient-centredness used, in many cases, to cop out from the real difficulties.

Here is my definition of patient-centredness for GPs. It is the ability and willingness to consider the patient as an equal in the communication, to seek out actively their preferences for involvement in decision making, and to ask about their ideas, concerns and expectations, and use these in the explanations, with an aim of reaching a shared understanding and possibly a shared management plan. This definition is enshrined in *The Consultation: an approach to learning and teaching* which was first published in 1984. The MRCGP consulting component, whose development started in 1990, is also framed round this definition. The current MRCGP merit criteria are in effect Tuckett *et al.*'s 'reactive explanation', from the book of their research published in 1985, famously called *Meetings between Experts*. The merit criteria are: that the doctor, while seeking the reason for the patient's attendance, explores their health beliefs; that in the explanation phase the doctor uses these elicited beliefs; and, thirdly, the doctor checks the patient's understanding. Tuckett's team found this 'reactive explanation' was a pretty rare bird, only seen in one in ten consultations, with a fairly loose definition, and one in 100, with a stricter definition. Nearly a decade earlier, Byrne and Long in their seminal work, *Doctors Talking to Patients*, had found much the same thing and were, to my knowledge, the first to define doctor- and patient-centredness.

So the fundamental question is how can you convert a rare bird into a common one? Improve the environment? Shoot the predators? Increase the food supply? The truth is that this is an odd rare bird, in that many from all walks of the profession and outside think that it is in fact common and talk about it as though they saw it every day. Only the true rare bird watcher knows they are wrong; they are seeing a 'Common Nice Mumble' and confusing it with the much rarer 'Lesser Spotted Empathy'. This is as far as this metaphor can usefully be stretched; the point is that patient-centred behaviour, however desired by well-meaning bodies, is unusual. I can say this with absolute certainty because I and over 100 trained colleagues have now watched over 30 000 consultations from over 4000 doctors, looking specifically for Tuckett et al.'s reactive explanation, and we have found that around 10% of doctors can demonstrate this behaviour regularly, which is what Tuckett and colleagues said more or less.

Now to my point about assessment. It takes time to produce a videotape of seven consultations that demonstrate the competencies required. Most registrars probably need to record at least five consultations for every one they submit. Say, 35 to 40 over a year, or less than one a week. Most trainers agree that there should be some review of consulting at least once a month, so say you submit your tape in the eighth month, you can have had at least seven sessions, watching say four or five at a time. There are, however, a number of trainers and registrars who object to this process, feeling the time could be better spent elsewhere, and that the preparation for summative assessment and the MRCGP somehow gets in the way of training. This group would advocate a quick simulation examination and so avoid the perceived tedious and unhelpful preparation. Who is right? Does assessment drive learning and, if it does, is it not reasonable to expect that a serious postgraduate examination needs practice and demonstrable expertise in the workplace to pass? When the MRCGP examination introduced a critical reading paper in the late 1980s, it was done to stimulate reading in registrars and subsequent research showed that it had the desired effect. The video examination was introduced to improve consulting; the evidence is that it is slowly having this effect – it would be a shame to back down now. Even those who would advocate a simple endpoint simulated examination must concede that to become a proficient consulter requires practice, intelligent feedback and more practice. Good consulting is truly skilful, like playing the piano well, and not many can do that without regular practice and tuition. General practice is currently the last refuge of the true generalist, and the major skill of the generalist is to really communicate and, to use Roger Neighbour's checkpoint, 'connect' with our patients. I have written about this too in my book, *The Doctor's Communication Handbook*, now in its fifth edition. This skill is not god given; most doctors do not possess it at the beginning of training, or even at the end – the assessments designed to measure this skill must encourage regular, rigorous performance review.

Let me finish on how to recognise the 'Lesser Spotted Empathy'. Empathy, as defined by the *Oxford English Dictionary*, is the power of identifying oneself with, and so fully comprehending, the person who is the subject of contemplation. How can doctors attempt to do this without eliciting our patients' ideas, concerns and expectations? To be truly empathetic that is what you have to do; currently only 10% can demonstrate this skill to a reasonable standard . . . it's not enough.

Chapter 4

What are we training for?

My registrar has just applied for extended training. This frightens me, and makes me feel more than usually inadequate as she has chosen to learn about forms of practising that I know little about; as her trainer I am likely to learn even more than she is. She has two motivations. One is to learn more about family medicine at the margins; she wishes to work with a parenting scheme to help disadvantaged mothers particularly develop skills of looking after their families; in so doing she will be closely involved with health visitors, social workers and community paediatricians. Her second motivation is to put off the evil day of actually doing general practice as currently constituted. But as I write this I slip into an Alice-type reverie; do I hear a bugle call? Could this be the seventh cavalry? Is that General Brown, with Colonel Milburn and dapper Lieutenant Chisholm? My heart leaps, saved she is in Yoda speak, but what's the name of that river nearby? Little Big what? I awake both elated and frightened, momentous deeds are afoot. A whole new contract is about to come into being, so no more 24-hour responsibility, apparently known in the negotiating trade as the John Wayne clause. Money following the patient, now where have I heard that before . . .? Money for quality, as defined in NSFs, but in realistic stages of attainment, but, and it is a big one, no more family doctor. You may feel that interpretation a little disingenuous, but no longer is Mrs Oddbody my patient; she is a patient of my practice. I will no longer have an individual long-term commitment to her wellbeing, or that of her family. My partners, registrars, assistants and practice nurses all share this responsibility. Yes, I hear you say, not really very different from the current situation in many practices, but it is different, fundamentally so. A whole value system has changed overnight, though it may take years for the effects to sink in. So back to the title of this article, what are we training for?

Well, let's start with what we needn't bother with. Continuity of care, previously a *sine qua non* of good general practice, enshrined in Professor John Howie's enablement measure of quality as judged by our patients, is not a priority any more. To remind you, the measure has three parts. How long the consultation lasts, how well the patient scores you on the enablement scale, and how well the patient knows you. After 30 years as a GP I know an awful lot of people, but most only a little; a few I know a lot about, a small proportion I know far too much about. This is the group that used to be friends till I learned about Fred with Lulu in the consulting room and then had to endure difficult parties pretending I didn't know. Will I no longer need to impart the skills of conversing with half-remembered people who think you know them well and who have trapped you in the toothpaste aisle at Tesco?

But wait, am I to lose my best excuse for sloppy consulting? Like many senior doctors having their consultations observed, when my registrar says to me, 'you are always telling me to know more about the patient as a person when they go out than when they come in, but I didn't see much of that this time' and I sanctimoniously reply, 'Ah but I already know them very well', when the reality is that I have the sketchiest knowledge of their life and none at all of their aspirations, beliefs and attitudes. You see, the reality that occurs to me is that without continuity I will have to consult better than I do now, because there will always be more that I need to know. Of course, good locums have known this for years; the bad ones just take the money and run, leaving you to repeat most of their encounters because of punter dissatisfaction. So we will have to teach the skills of one-off consulting and, just maybe, we should be teaching it more effectively than we seem to be doing with serial consulting. We could retreat further into the Victorian medical model and persist with the horribly entrenched and communicatively disastrous 'history taking'.

To consult well takes time; this is now unarguable, say Freeman *et al.*,[1] though I could argue just a bit. A good consulter will do more with the time than a poor one; many can achieve in ten minutes what a disorganised consulter has not achieved in 20, and this is of course too subtle for most research. A quality marker has been that longer consultations contain more health promotion; well hallelujah, but just a small dose of caution here. When the MRCGP examination piloted the consulting skills criteria, we found health promotion by doctors to be a destructive process in many if not most cases because, to trained GP observers, the doctor's agenda effectively swamped that of the patient. To earn lots in our new contract, we will need to practise this skill daily; more and more time for my NSF quality standard agenda and less and less for what the patient actually came about. This, of course, may be good ultimately for the 'health of the nation', though not its exchequer . . . time will tell, but not in my lifetime I suspect.

So what am I to train for? Good investigative consulting and patient advocacy, or protocol-based consulting with cash at the end of it? 'Oh come on Pete', you are saying, 'that's a bit over the top; quality is quality; there is a good evidence base and we are going to have to teach effective consulting that achieves both agendas'. Well maybe, but where is the evidence that we doctors are particularly good at either variety of consulting? And we can't escape from the figures relating to compliance/concordance/adherence with medical advice, which remain low. Of course, if I don't know Mrs Oddbody well, which in this new world I won't, I have less incentive to listen to her and more to inform her. This is the situation now with cervical screening, and we all know how much informed consent there is in that endeavour. Previous *BMJ*s have railed about that, especially the one with the tangoing couple on the front of September 99. Type 'Joan Austoker' into Google and see what comes out.

David Misselbrook, another GP educator, has written a clever book, full of long words and frighteningly erudite quotations, called *Thinking about Patients*.[2] He says that we need to rediscover what it is to be a healer; he reminds us that our role is to parent rarely, fix sometimes, translate often and listen always. He wonders who will win the struggle for power between doctor, patient and politician. I am not awarding any prizes for the answer.

My friend and hero, David Pendleton, gave a talk to the RCGP Spring Meeting in Birmingham in April; he talked of trust and values. I quote him verbatim.

> *In order to be trusted, professionals need to demonstrate four attributes. First, there is competence. It is almost impossible to trust any professional whose competence is in question. Second, there is care. We are more likely to be trusted by people for whom we care. Third, there is consistency. Trust is enhanced by consistent demonstration of the same standards, values and attitudes. Finally, there is courage. In our professional lives we occasionally need to take a stand. Those who can stand up to pressure with a little courage will prove to be more worthy of our trust. Scientia and caritas are reflected in the first two attributes, but they may be insufficient without consistency and courage. . . . Direction emerges from values in action and a careful analysis of what is required to give them life. Purpose, vision and values are a mix of head and heart, of evidence and conviction, of thought and feeling. So is general practice.*

He went on to point out that in the cut-throat world of business those organisations with clearly stated values did better.

So what are the values of tomorrow's GPs to be? Who will decide these values? At present, it looks like the politicians to me. Will the RCGP be brave and take up the challenge to state the values for the next generation of doctors? I hope they do and then I will know what I am training for.

References

1 Freeman GK, Horder JP, Howie JGR *et al.* (2002) Evolving general practice consultation in Britain: issues of length and context. *British Medical Journal.* **324**: 880–2.
2 Misselbrook D (2001) *Thinking about Patients.* Petroc Press: Newbury.

Chapter 5

Hypertension: a tutorial for our time

Have you 'done' hypertension with your registrar lately? How many sessions did it take and what angles did you cover, I wonder? I write this while feeling a surge of unease about the whole direction of Western medicine. My favourite columnist, the *BMJ*'s Minerva, mentioned she was feeling this way and wondered if all was a vast con trick led by the vested interests of the huge pharmaceutical companies. Her suggested antidote was a trip to Phil Hammond's road show. In this particular *BMJ* there was another article from the Little *et al.* paper factory, discussing how difficult it is to get an accurate blood pressure reading, that surgery readings are far too high, ambulatory may be a bit better, but best of all is a series of readings produced at home by the patient from those machines advertised with nose hair removal gadgets in the *Innovations* catalogue or such like. I have always felt that possession of such a machine was a sure sign of introverted hypochondria characterised by an internal locus of control nearing the top of the scale. My father, a GP too, held a similar view about thermometers, and stamped on as many as he could. I have sometimes wondered about the levels of mercury in the older population of South Shields, thank heavens it wasn't mercury sphygs that he took a dislike to.

Hypertension, we doctors are taught, is an asymptomatic risk factor. It is not an illness and it is definitely not a disease. But try telling that to our patients, they just don't and never will believe us. To the average patient hypertension is a bodily reality. They can feel it. This of course goes some of the way to explaining the dismal figures on compliance/concordance/ adherence with hypertensive treatment. The truth is most of us take drugs if we think it is important enough and we have a clear rationale in our minds. Patients know when their blood pressure is up, they feel hypertensive, and on those days they take the tablets. If they feel relaxed, on holiday, etc., well it's obvious that treatment is not needed. This 'logic' drives statistically framed clinicians daft. It's all in the framing, you see; doctors are taught a complex mathematically based rationale, founded in actuarial tables and EBM, for 'treating' the risk that is hypertension. They adhere to expert produced protocols, consult learned tables and computer models, and decide that treatment may reduce the probability of an event by a certain percentage that might be advantageous to the individual patient. To the individual, of course, if the doctor thinks they need treatment they must be ill. Now I am not going to bore you with zillions of references but if you want some I will email them to you, all I am now going to say has as good an evidence base as any other medical fact. The diagnosis of hypertension is not good for the individual patient. Walking into the surgery fit and then being told that my BP is up to treatable levels immediately doubles the odds of me having panic attacks, my sickness rate also doubles and I immediately cut down my participation in sport. My incidence of impotence shoots up, if you see what I mean. This is all before I start on whatever cocktail of drugs the latest protocol has in store for me and their attendant side effects. So this is a harmful diagnosis. Have we yet got a computer model that works out how much good we have to do with our treatment to outweigh the harm we have already done?

I am steeped in hypertension, if that makes sense. As a practice we joined the MRC mild hypertension trial in the late 1970s, along with 170 or so other practices and 17 354 patients, and continued in various stages for over a decade. I came to know and love the cumbersome heavyweight random zero sphygmomanometer, though a partner, perhaps wiser than me, still managed to record every BP as 140/90. The screening caravan in the car park (donated by Merck, Sharp and Dohme Ltd) was there so long that it sank into the tarmac. Eventually all this labour and endeavour was written up (Mild hypertension – is there pressure to treat? Cambridge University Press 1987) and what did we learn?

Well, to begin with that mild hypertension was not much of an isolated risk, in fact in middle-aged women it was not really a risk at all; that if you smoked then taking beta-blockers for blood pressure was a waste of time; and that long-term bendrofluazide, at the then correct dose of 5 mg, was more dangerous than the risk from blood pressure because of hypokalaemia. The trial did reduce the incidence of strokes but not the all-causes mortality, and had no significant effect on coronary heart disease. We also learned that the famous drug 'placebo' controlled 40% of men and 45% of women. It was during this time that I attended a training day on taking blood pressures; in a large room we were played a recording of Korotkov's sounds and asked to record the blood pressure. This was a room of trained health professionals and the results were a widely based normal curve. Even though we all heard the same thing, we recorded worryingly large differences. This has haunted me since. More recently a keen hypertensively minded partner bought two top-of-the-range electronic machines to improve our care of diabetic hypertensives. We tested them on the staff and against our ageing and environmentally dangerous mercury machines. The two machines produced different results by approximately 15 mm of mercury, the lowest reader was still on average 5 mm higher than our mercury ones. Almost everyone was at least mildly hypertensive as judged by the top machine. I remember wet Sundays of my childhood being happily filled by the pungent smelling painting-by-numbers kits and here am I nearly in my second childhood less happily treating by numbers. I know there are impressive trials, much expense and an array of dedicated well-informed 'experts' driving this huge hypertension bandwagon, but is this whole edifice really a flickering mirage? This faint and distorted image is made up of fundamentally inaccurate and volatile measurements mixed with a nervous and uncomprehending patient base, and at least I could hang my paintings on the wall.

Now to the old hobbyhorse of communication. What do we tell patients? Well some professionals of my local acquaintance tell patients to make urgent appointments with their doctors because their blood pressure is dangerously high, at 145/95. Nasty little caravans in the centre of town advertising cholesterol testing are particularly prone to this and other similar crimes, but even worse are the 'fitness' gyms. But what about me? Am I perfect? No I am confused, half caught up in this tenuous belief system and half non-believer facing patients who mostly want the decisions to be simple, logical and unequivocal. I start talking about NNTs or 1000 patient years and try to pull myself together with PPBs (personal probability of benefit stats, an acronym coined by David Misselbrook). The MRC trial PPB for 100–109 diastolic range in 35–64 year olds over five years was 175 to 1. Most of us would not consider a bet on a horse at such silly odds. If I am older, the odds drop sometimes to 20 to 1. Have you met anyone that regularly made money on horses priced at 20 to 1? Underneath all of this is the anxiety that I started this column with. Shouldn't we be doing something better for our patients, and the exchequer, than overfeeding them dubious medications on the off chance that the odd one of them, entirely unknown to them or me, might just live a little longer than they might otherwise have done? Can't we start nationwide happy classes or something similar, a search for a purpose within our society rather than eking out our days medicalised, fearful of death and introspective of our health? There has to be more worth to our lives than that.

Chapter 6

A retrospective look into the future

I have handed in my badge. It's not training that has taken its toll, but the old get up and go has got up and gone. My gorgeous registrar, the last of a long line (18 in fact, plus a stint at course organising), took me out for lunch last week. She is young, just married, and actually wants to be a GP. This pleases me. In fact the vast majority of my ex-registrars or trainees, as most were, are practising GPs. In addition, there are a couple of child psychiatrists, a dermatologist and a public health physician. Only one has not got the MRCGP qualification; she never got round to it and is one of the child psychiatrists. Not one of the 17 failed. This also pleases me.

There is still a considerable dislike of the examination in some circles. Of course this is not new, and even my own father in the early 1970s had little time for it. But the people who dislike it now are different from those of 25 years ago. Now it is a disaffected cadre of educators, including the odd Director of my experience, who have a visceral dislike of its perceived effect on the training experience and a diffuse dislike of its methodology. The present crop of registrars quite like it, judging from the findings of research published in this journal,[1] and are certainly taking it in vast numbers, currently increasing by about 150 a year. I had better declare an interest at this point. I am the Convenor of the Examination, and have been an examiner since 1981, so I am biased.

Going back to looking back, what are registrars like now compared with my first registrar in 1976, or even me in 1972? There are of course more similarities than differences. The greatest difference is in pay and conditions. Registrars are now, in relative terms, richer and work far less hard than they did. I know there will be exceptions to this sweeping statement, but very few do much on call anymore, most are earning £40,000 or more and when finished can easily command £70,000 a year by doing regular but not too onerous locum work. This is a good time to be young in medicine, but it is perhaps not such a good time to be at the other end of one's career, either as a partner or as a consultant. There is the gender effect. Women have dominated the training schemes for some time, and the hours have been feminised, as has the commitment. The traditional male model of general practice is all but dead. Continuity of care is going through its last spasmodic dying twitches, and obscure hidden formulae are to guide our future pay and workload. At least in the last few years a few people understood the *Red Book*, but the new developments make this state of affairs much fairer, as now no one understands them.

'Quality' is much bandied about as the Holy Grail to be searched for. The trouble is, of course, the myriad of definitions of quality, some clearly Orwellian Newspeak, usually emanating from a central organisation like the Department of Health, or the disciplinarian from the likes of the GMC, or the union view from the BMA or the academic from the Royal College. The MRCGP, for all its faults, and it is bound to have some, does try to look at reasonable and contemporary definitions of quality emanating from workaday practice, and by setting such a syllabus ensures that registrars are at least measured against a notional standard derived from the profession at a crucial staging post in their careers.

How does it do this? Most importantly by the constitution of the panel of examiners, currently 150 or more, representing all parts of the UK and all in active practice. This is an inbuilt reality check on the content of the examination. Very few of the panel are in academic departments, but the vast majority are trainers or have partners who are. They are selected for aptitude – the ability to assess is not synonymous with the ability to teach – and then further intensive training follows to get up to speed with the various modules.

Critics of the examination cite issues of reliability and validity. The examination is remarkably reliable considering the level of sophisticated and complex human behaviour that it attempts to measure in its oral and consulting components. The Americans are far slicker with their huge testing organisations and impressive reliability statistics, but take a quick look behind the scenes and you will see that the testing is of a much less sophisticated level of behaviour than we are attempting. We are trying to test the real useful working knowledge and skills of a human being from the top 2% of our educational system, who has been through five years of university education and then at least four more postgraduate years of supposedly intensive training. There is a major problem with reliability, as it is quite easy to be reliably wrong as well as right – just listen to the pub bore. This is the validity argument, which is like beauty often being in the eye of the beholder. In the 1980s, when university courses mushroomed throughout the Western world, it was possible, in all seriousness, to spend several years studying hamburgerology (yes, an -ology), and in terms of validity this could be viewed as a high-quality purveyor of a low-quality product. A shudder runs down the spine at the faint and fleeting thought that the MRCGP might be becoming similar – a high-quality measure of a low-quality product. Now I don't really believe this, but I am worried. Today's registrar is better educated, better read and in general a better consulter than they would have been 25 years ago. However, they are less practical and do not have any depth to their experience. The Postgraduate Medical Education and Training Board (PMETB) is arriving soon, with the 'Standards' extracted from its original name, the SHO review suggests a not unreasonable form of rolling accreditation, and use of the word 'assessment' in this context is frowned upon. There is strong pressure to lower all the hurdles to summative assessment levels, 2–4%, as failure cannot be countenanced politically, so where does the exam fit for future registrars? The honest truth is that I don't know, but we need a debate on it, and quickly. Some directors don't see a place, while others see it as a crucial end-point measure of general medical competence – a star to which to hitch your wagon. My registrars wanted to be measured against a standard that was attainable but not easy, and that marked them as reasonably competent in their chosen field. In this brave new world of rolling portfolios, 360-degree appraisals and patient satisfaction measures, none of which I denigrate, we are still going to have to be sure that we have doctors who know some medicine, who appreciate the ethical minefield in which we work and, most crucially, who can apply this knowledge effectively in the consulting room.

The current examination is strong on knowledge and communication, but needs the development of a true clinical component. This might be undertaken in conjunction with Deaneries. The definitions of the appropriate skills need to be agreed, as does the timing of the measuring. This argument relates to the production of a training curriculum for general practice, which has been much discussed but not decided on yet. Who knows whether there will be a Part 1 and Part 2? It is certainly not for me to say. My job is to implement what my bosses, the RCGP Council, tell me to do. What I do know is that Registrars don't want a devalued currency, so whatever does come out of curricula, reviews and restructuring, there must be a qualification in there somewhere to be aimed for, and which opens doors that are not accessible to those without it. This is a competitive world, and now I spend more time being a patient than a doctor I want my doctors to be seen to be competent and to have had their metal tested by a modern, wide-ranging assessment that still embraces the concept of failure. In doing so I also hope that if the assessment maintains or even improves a standard, so will the profession. Mediocrity is to be fought at all costs.

Reference

1 Dixon H (2003) Candidates' views of the MRCGP examination. *Educ Prim Care.* **14**: 146–57.

Chapter 7

Mabel: an anecdote

In the spirit of narrative-based medicine here is a genuinely true story, especially the ending, to make a change.

When she was young, she loved horses. Men were incidental and her job at the Post Office only an interruption between the visits to the stable and the companionship of her beloved horse, Elley. The day Elley died, part of Mabel died too; she never found a replacement.

Age withered and rumpled Mabel: the bags under her eyes were spectacular, her jowls hung like a bloodhound and her chin folded like a well-used fan. The bottom eyelids began to fold outwards in this general collapse of the flesh, giving her a doleful doggy look that was both sad and a little macabre. By 70 she was heroically ugly: 16 stone with osteoarthritis of her hips and rapidly deforming hands, the knuckles swelling and the fingers falling sideways. She lived in a little council flat in the old centre of the town. When I became her GP, Mabel had not set foot out of the door for five years; she was 72.

Here was I, fresh from general practice training, green as grass, an idealist in a long tradition of young medics. I was going to sweep away the inefficiencies of my older colleagues. I would diagnose people, find all the diseases others had missed; I was going to make people better. Every surgery was an exciting challenge, every visit an adventure. It was a Thursday in October when I was first called to visit Mabel. The message on my page gave the reason as 'legs'.

The entrance to her flat was obscure and it took several minutes to find it. It was the lady in the health food shop who put me out of my misery.

'You the doctor come for Mabel?'

I nodded self-consciously, carrying my overlarge new plastic doctor's bag and red stethoscope. She was a large no-nonsense lady blocking the doorway of her mysterious smelling shop. She pointed to an alleyway.

'Down there, she's on the right. Take her her vitamins every week I do. Funny old trout really.'

She looked at me properly with a squinting assessment.

'You're the new doctor? Gawd you don't look old enough to deliver newspapers.'

She smiled.

'Good luck anyway.'

(Ah those were the days!)

Mabel's door was ajar, a smell emanated, which I did not recognise then, but has become familiar to me over the years as that of human bodies past their best. The room was dark, curtains half-drawn, and there by the gas fire sat Mabel. I say sat but this is a totally inadequate description. I don't think that there is a word in the English language to truly describe Mabel's posture. She was slumped in the chair as if she had just fallen backwards into it; her vast blue legs were apart revealing a highly inadequate gusset. Sharon Stone she wasn't. She made an effort to focus on me, without any change in position.

'Who the f*** are you?'

I was unprepared for this greeting. I stumbled over an object, became unbalanced because of my heavy cumbersome bag, staggered dangerously towards Mabel's open crotch, stabilised myself just in time and mumbled unconvincingly.

'I am Dr Tate, the new doctor from the health centre.'

She looked at me with withering disbelief. I discovered an early truth: people in their own houses have much more power than in my surgery. I was on Mabel's territory and she was boss. I was uncomfortable. There was a silence. I picked out a stale urine smell emanating from the chair and warmed by the gas fire. My eyes started to water. I couldn't think of what to say, I was not in control. Mabel gestured with frighteningly deformed hands to what seemed to be her exposed nether regions.

'Me legs,' she said.

Silence fell again. I looked at her legs more closely. Below her knees on both legs were large ulcerated areas. The legs were massive. She was wearing slippers but no socks. I knelt down to get a closer look. The carpet squelched and my knees immediately felt damp. My senior partner's warning came to mind too late.

'Off to see Mabel, are you? Well, you had better learn the rules quickly. Rule one: never sit down and never kneel down. Rule two: never forget the first rule.'

I just had. While this unpleasant realisation was literally sinking in, my eyes, now more accustomed to the gloom could focus on the ulcers. They were huge, at least 6" by 6", they were covered in a yellow foul-smelling pus, and, no surely not, there was movement. There were maggots. A wave of nausea hit me, I gagged and fought desperately against vomiting over Mabel's urine- and pus-enriched carpet.

That was the first time; all I saw then was a deformed maggot-infested old crone who repulsed me. General practice was not going to be too much fun if there were many Mabels.

I was wrong, Mabel continued to teach me and over the months we became accustomed to each other; 'friends' would be the wrong word, but Mabel thought she needed me and I became fascinated by her story. In fact, the district nurses heroically dressed and coped with her ulcers, the social services department set up an efficient care package. They got her up in the morning, meals on wheels ('muck in a truck' according to Mabel) fed her, the nurse assistant bed-bathed her regularly and someone came to put her to bed.

My role as her doctor was very peripheral but to Mabel crucial. To Mabel, I was what stood between her and the great reaper. To me, I wasn't sure what to do; medical school hadn't really equipped me for this long-term pastoral sort of care. I had been taught to *do* things, so I did – I fiddled with her tablets. Someone years ago had diagnosed an underactive thyroid gland, so, as she was always tired and sluggish, as well as being enormously overweight, I put the dose of thyroxin up to get things going. This gave me something to ask about when I visited. 'Was there any improvement?' She teased me by offering glimmers of hope, 'a little better doctor, but my bowels are bad'. So, I gave her bowel mixture. My therapeutic courage began to rise; I experimented with diuretics to release the fluid trapped in her bloated body. Her heart was a bit irregular so I tried digoxin, a heart stimulant, known for centuries and extracted from the foxglove plant. I felt like a real doctor, I was doing something for this unfortunate old lady. By this stage Mabel had me visiting her once a week. A ritual was developing; the care assistant had left a teapot ready and two cups. I boiled the tea, examined Mabel while it brewed, and had a quick cup while Mabel told me stories of the past, nearly always related to horses. The encounter would finish with me writing a new prescription for my latest experiment and telling her it was my greatest wish that one day she would be able to go to the chemist to get these herself.

After a while the ritual changed a little, she began giving me presents. Old cameras, not expensive ones, tatty old Kodak box cameras. I used to try and refuse them but she was insistent; a level of guilt began to build up in me; in the end I used to pop into the Red Cross shop across the road with each new acquisition. Then new things were produced: hideous plastic shoehorns with antlers, tacky leather bookmarks, little chrome picture frames, etc. The guilt level rose even more; Mabel was buying these things via an intermediary just to keep me coming regularly. Didn't she know I would come anyway, I said to myself? As the realisation of my importance to Mabel's existence really began to impinge on my conscience, I vowed to try to do more with my professional influence. I set a goal in my mind: I would mobilise Mabel. I would get her out of that ghastly little room for a walk in the truly fresh air.

Now every encounter finished not just with a wish but a goal, to walk across the room and back, to walk into the back yard, etc. She began to respond; a frame was conjured up by the nurses who also became excited by this vision of a mobile Mabel. We professionals now aimed our whole therapeutic force into getting Mabel to go out; it gave us a purpose. I began leading her by the hand across her sticky carpet. The presents stopped but her humour improved. A few years fell away, a light returned to the eyes; she talked of her beloved Elley. For the first time I could actually see her, blonde hair streaming, galloping across the Downs. This ruined old lady had been young, vivacious, even attractive, once.

Then came the day. A domiciliary physiotherapist had been working with Mabel for some weeks and was convinced that she was ready to try a little journey. As she told me this standing in Mabel's back yard, I noticed she was clutching a large plastic shoehorn with antlers. Mabel greeted me enthusiastically:

'I am going to bloody do it.'

She waited for a reaction; I just smiled and nodded.

'Tomorrow I'm going up the road to the naffing Post Office for me pension. Worked there for 20 year, don't suppose anyone will know me now.'

She mused and continued.

'That nice girl thinks I should do it so I will.'

She looked at me and I realised that I was not important any more, that was why the presents had stopped. I should have been happy but a little touch of pique entered my soul. Doctors need to be important.

The next morning, while I was seeing patients in my morning surgery, I received an emergency call. Would I go immediately to Abingdon Post Office. My patient Mabel Crump had been involved in a serious accident; the ambulance men were standing by. I hate leaving a full surgery; it ruins the day and makes me very tense. I already knew in my own mind that Mabel had slipped off her frame, twisted her ankle or similar and that this would turn out to be a fuss about nothing. I was irritated too by the feeling that this was my own fault anyway by encouraging this unwise excursion.

I arrived at the scene in an unhelpful frame of mind. There was a large crowd outside the Post Office, where the ambulance was parked with its blue light flashing. There was another crowd about 50 yards down the road. I parked my car behind the ambulance waving my stethoscope at the policeman to identify myself. (A friend of mine did that once while speeding to an emergency, the policeman waved the handcuffs back.) I have to point out that at this time doctors were still required at the scene of accidents. Though it has to be said that most doctors' training and experience in emergency medicine was not too good. My experience of a busy London casualty department and a spell as a ship's doctor equipped me better than most, but this experience soon rusted without the regular refresher courses that I didn't go to.

I did not need any experience here, Mabel was dead. She was lying on the pavement, flat on her back, head in a pool of blood and legs characteristically splayed apart. Her eyes were wide and staring, though the expression seemed more of wonder than of horror.

'What happened?' I said inadequately.

'Run over by a horse,' said the large, matter-of-fact ambulanceman.

'Sorry, say that again.'

'Yes, a bloody runaway horse hit her fair and square; look at her frame.' He pointed at a mangled piece of aluminium tubing some feet away.

'Didn't do the bloody horse any good either, vet's just shot it.'

He gestured to the other gathering down the road. A wave of sadness and of uselessness engulfed me, mingled with a feeling that this was just too unbelievable to be true. Five years and she never went out, the first time she does she is run over by a bolting horse in the centre of a little market town where there are no horses.

I felt a hand touch my sleeve; it was the lady from the health food shop.

'Come with me Doc, I want to show you something.'

The ambulance men took Mabel away to the post-mortem room as a favour to the police whose job it was technically. The butcher took the horse away. I was led into Mabel's flat.

'The lady at the Post Office said that Mabel screamed "Elley" just before the horse hit her. I think she thought her old horse had come back for her. May be she was right. Here, look here.'

She pulled open a large drawer to reveal bottles of pills going back several years, all unopened.

'She didn't believe in pills.'

She looked at me pityingly.

'Did you like your shoehorn?'

Chapter 8

The ICE man cometh:
a painful tutorial

In 1979, three Thames Valley course organisers, Theo Schofield, Peter Havelock and myself, plus our new friend, social psychologist David Pendleton, first used the triumvirate of Ideas, Concerns and Expectations (ICE) as the basis of understanding our patients' health beliefs, and started to include this concept in our day-release teaching. This led to the book, *The Consultation*, an approach to learning and teaching.[1] We have a new book out any minute now with a very similar message.[2] Over the years, ICE has perhaps become an overused mnemonic, trotted out with little meaning by many hoping to please teachers and examiners. It is time to redress the balance.

You see, I am recovering from a severe attack of ideas, concerns and expectations. This relates to the fact that I have also been a bit poorly. Those of you who don't like illness stories will perhaps stop reading now, but let me try to persuade you to bear with me. My first idea was that I was too fat (17 stone), I was concerned about my nagging angina-like pain, previously but dubiously diagnosed as oesophagitis, and I expected weight loss would make me feel better and perhaps improve the gout too. Having tried every conventional diet in the books, to no avail, the low-carbohydrate strategy seemed worth a try. It worked a treat. Within two weeks a youthful feeling returned, the gout went, as did the 'angina', and a stone fell off. A life appeared ahead and the future beckoned. Ah, *hubris*, always just around the corner. Unfortunately, I have sick sinus syndrome and have been paced since 1977. Wires are fragile things, with limited life-spans, and difficult to remove. By the time of this saga I had four: three broken ones and a live one connected to the current box. One was 'tied off' below the skin in the upper right breast. This was no real problem as there was plenty of fat to cushion it – indeed Mae West might have been envious – but as the fat evaporated the wire began poking through the skin. What to do? There was a learned fear of cardiologists from 25 years of interventions and different opinions. Idea: it's a breast problem, get a nice plastic surgeon to snip the wire, easy. Done, a quick day case and no fuss. Down to 14 stone now, more energetic than for a decade and the little grey cells bubbling away with a vigour now freed from the custard of lethargy that had seemed to be engulfing them. But what are these night sweats and funny feelings in the chest? Over eight weeks of increasing lethargy and ineffective self-treatment the concern is clear. I know I have an infected wire, but I also know that to treat me properly they will have to take the whole lot out, and this is not an attractive prospect. Eventually my registrar takes the decision for me. She tells me I will be dead if something is not done soon and checks the CRP, which comes back at 219 (normal <8). Paradoxically, this makes me feel better as it proves I am not skiving. My ideas are that this will be a long job, my concerns are that I won't make it, and my expectations are of an extremely unpleasant few weeks.

Let me say that everyone, from the cleaner to the consultant cardiologist, was kind beyond the call of duty, but implacable, all of them. They put an IV line in, warned me of six weeks' treatment and said I probably had endocarditis and that first and foremost the old pacing system had to come out. Now as you know, I write books on doctor/patient communication, so I tried some patient/doctor communication. 'What is it going to be like to take the old wires out?', I enquired. 'Think of it as legalised GBH', said my fellow Geordie SR, with a smile. This honesty quieted me somewhat, '. . . er, what about the risks?'. 'Ah, only for old ladies. Of course there is tamponade, but the R ventricle is such a low-pressure system it's no real problem', came the reply. The insouciance of it all. There was no point in whingeing.

'. . . er, the pain?', I ventured. 'We'll give you what the Russkis gave the Chechens, that'll keep you quiet.' Well it did, and with added fentanyl, a five-hour struggle felt like 45 minutes. Vaguely remembered feelings of tugging and the heart mildly objecting to being turned inside out were academic rather than emotional. I did, however, sort of get the feeling that all was not 100%.

'Well, how did it go?', say I brightly the next day to assembled band at foot of bed. Brief but unmistakable dropping of eyelids, shuffling and strained smiles ensued. 'Fine, just fine.' There is a strained attempt at humour. 'Shame your scrap value has collapsed.' And my friend the Geordie is detailed to come back with a slightly fuller version of the truth.

'We thought we might lose you, you know', is the opening gambit. 'I thought only old ladies died?' 'Well, yes, of tamponade, but it was the IVC (intravascular coagulation) that really worried us.' 'Eh?' 'Well, like toxic shock, all those wires with toxins on them being stripped off, too much and it all coagulates and that's it really.' My ideas on informed consent were shaken to the core. Was I pleased I didn't know this risk beforehand? I decided that yes, I was, and sank further into passivity. In the lull that followed, the SR filled the gap. 'Shame the wire snapped.' I felt like a stunned trout and let the fly dangle in front of me. 'You see, there's a fragment we will need to take out.' 'Where?' was the best I could manage. 'Oh, it's just in the pulmonary artery, no real problem. We had better put you on fragmin (blood thinner) injections till we fish it out. The interventional radiologists are going to do it next week.' So that was all right then. My ideas about fragments of wire in pulmonary arteries were vague in the extreme, my concerns were also vague but much nastier and my expectations of more pain and faffing about 100% accurate. 'Fragment' turned out to be a euphemism for 2.5 inches of something that looked like barbed wire, but was in fact a very frayed 25-year-old wire. I felt inexplicably better for it being out.

'Is that it?' The eyelids drop again. My concernometer registers 'Oh shit' on a five-point scale. 'Well, there is another fragment . . . stuck in the right ventricle . . . would need open heart surgery . . . probably OK to leave it.' Now 'probably' is a word for doctors, it is not a good word for patients, but the repartee has dried up. The SR fills the silence. 'Your creatinine is not too good, too much gentamicin, so we will have to keep an eye on the renal failure first anyway.' Kidney failure and nasty fragments somewhere crucial? A Chagall-like vision of dead daffy-looking ducks floated by and the concernometer went off the scale, but no real sound came out other than a sort of John Mills 1945 propaganda film: 'Oh, that's a bit of a bugger, ah well . . .' I am reminded of Kenneth Williams' famous rejoinder to the question, 'Dammit man, where is your stiff upper lip?'. 'Above this loose, flabby chin.'

Weeks went by, and I was allowed home to give the IV antibiotics myself, much to the chagrin of the wonderful nurses who were all firmly of the opinion that most doctors could not be trusted to wipe their noses, let alone do complicated injections. I felt better too. Shame about the angina, which had recurred on mild exertion, but my spirits were up and I was not dead, the agonising gout had gone as the kidney function had improved, and the thought of going back to general practice, my patients and partners was an attractive one. Repeated echocardiograms showed no vegetations, but the tricuspid valve was damaged, and my relative lack of fitness was ascribed to this. 'Get fit' was the message, so I did and within four weeks was walking the fells and the Roman Wall at Housesteads for 10 miles on a Saturday in January in −5°C with no angina to speak of. A check treadmill was arranged for the week before going back to work, but that was just crossing the Ts. I felt good, no pacemaker for the first time for 25 years and soon this would all be over and just a story, my concernometer had dropped to zero and my expectations were of a busy return. Did I mention *hubris*?

Even I could see the ST segments were very wonky, the chest tightness was mild and I did do nine minutes, but the eyelids were down again. The consultant came and was solicitous and firm, 'looks like stents . . . need angiography PDQ . . . in fact have a cancellation, see you tomorrow'.

The ideas about stents are pretty good, could be worse, and the new antibiotic ones seem a real step forward. The concerns that it might just be a bit dodgy are not too bad and the expectations of still getting back to work soon are OK. Another trip through the hospital on my back, and I swear I could navigate this hospital just by looking at the ceilings. Much bonhomie is followed by silence again, the television shows a picture I don't want to see. Why is there very little white dye getting down that big artery on the left ventricle? 'Peter, I am afraid you have a problem. . .' says the kind and slightly sad voice. Stenting is not possible, there is critical occlusion of the left main coronary artery (all that red wine to no avail), and the right system is not too good to boot. I was fairly fit half an hour ago, now I am an invalid facing another major heart operation, with all the uncertainties that entails. He won't even let me go home because the narrowing is so critical. Bleating about walking the Roman Wall is to no avail. 'Peter, which cardiac surgeon would you like?' Being a GP, I know who I don't like, and coded responses pass between us. He smiles and says he would recommend the youngest, who is a good communicator. A further smile, almost a wink; this suits me fine, but being a patient I want him to be the best operator in the UK and don't really care if he is ruder than Sir Lancelot Spratt. Ah, how values change. So here I am writing this three weeks post quadruple CABG and open heart surgery to remove the offending fragment, which was apparently not doing me any good. So the chest surgery could be construed as lucky, in a perverse sort of way. I am afraid my ideas, concerns and expectations are still a bit wobbly, they haven't settled from the operation yet. I think the expectations are the hardest things at the moment, but I will report back, God willing.

References

1 Schofield T, Havelock P and Tate P (1984) *The Consultation*. Oxford University Press: Oxford.
2 Schofield T, Havelock P and Tate P (2003) *The New Consultation*. Oxford University Press: Oxford.

Chapter 9

Making a difference

This article is for those of you who have just struggled through an endless evening surgery, are worried about your forthcoming appraisal, don't know where you are going to find the time for the series of critical incident meetings your PCT are insisting on, and are now slumped in the armchair at home wondering if it is all worth it. I am here to tell you that it is. It has taken me some odd routes to find this out and sadly it is a truism that you have to stop doing something to discover how valuable it was. I have retired from active general practice after 30 years because of a spot of bother with the old ticker. Since this decision leaked out I have been inundated with letters, phone calls and sometimes embarrassingly emotional embraces by the broccoli in Tesco's. My official retirement date was 01.8.03 and to date (it is the 17 August today) I have accumulated over 200 cards and letters. I am not writing this to boast, hubris is too unforgiving for that, and I am well aware that many of Harold Shipman's patients thought he was wonderful, but I wanted to share some of the sentiments that have been expressed to make you think and cheer you up.

Here is a letter from a young man in his mid-20s, I have known him for 10 years and he has struggled with severe psychological problems, with an intrinsic severe depressive element. He wished to study psychology at university so that he could both understand himself better and in so doing help others with similar afflictions. I both listened to him and encouraged him, but really felt I was just a bit player in his theatre of life. He wrote:

> I have regretfully been informed that you have retired recently. You have been my doctor for many years and a suitable replacement capable of filling your shoes will be hard to find. For me, the two most important things in life are to have no regrets (if possible) and to make a difference. In my darkest times you were there for me and you made a difference to my life. At present, I am in my second year at university and my battle, although never-ending, is becoming easier. I wouldn't have gotten this far without your understanding and care. I will always be in your debt.

*I sincerely wish you a happy retirement, you will be sorely missed.
Many thanks Doctor.*

Another letter from a long-standing patient set me musing about the true
doctor–patient relationship. You may be aware that I have written books
and oodles of articles on the subject but never got to the inner kernel.
Tony had his first heart attack while playing the clarinet in 1975 and I
persuaded him much against his will to go into hospital. He is still going,
but now with an implantable defibrillator. He used to boast his was bigger
than mine as I only had a puny pacemaker. Tony loved telling me awful
jokes, partly to cover his very real fear of doctors and death. He wrote:

> *It is with mixed emotions that I write, having just learned of your
> retirement due to recent health problems. Mixed emotions, relief that
> you have survived a pretty nasty setback to your health and sadness that
> it is unlikely that our paths will cross again and that I have no-one to
> tell those awful jokes to, and gratitude for your concern about my health
> over the last 25 years.*
>
> *I like to think that we enjoyed something more than a doctor–patient
> relationship, but I think that most of your patients felt the same, which
> is a testament to your caring person. You are indeed a credit to your
> profession. PS Did you hear the one about . . . ?*

Tony, like many patients who I knew well, had a close relationship in one
sense and a distant one in another. We were friends, but only so far as his
life impinged on my professional responsibility to him. We both knew a
little about each other's life, would not go to the pub together, but would
smile and chat briefly if we met in one. You can't become too friendly with
patients because the relationship is essentially a service one. Most doctors
learn early in their career that getting too close to patients is professionally
unwise and often leads to hurt, on both sides, and a lingering fractured
friendship in a small community can be quite a millstone.

Sometimes we forget what we do. When I opened the next letter I
couldn't place the name, the face or even the sex of the writer. After some
research I now can, she is a 35-year-old lady who normally saw another
partner but saw me two or three times when her own doctor was away.
She wrote:

> *As you are aware, I went through a difficult period last year with the
> break-up of my marriage and I reached an all-time low. The genuinely
> sensitive manner in which you dealt with the problems that I had at
> that time made a major difference to me. Occasionally we arrive at a*

juncture in our lives where we are faced with stark choices. I have no doubt in my mind that your help was a significant factor in enabling me to make the right choice, and I am very grateful for your help.

Try as I might, I can't recall the encounters but I must have done something right. When my father died aged 58, a GP too, I had to clear out his damp basement surgery in South Shields. There was the Monarch of the Glens on the wall doing battle with the peeling wallpaper, and there was his examination couch stacked high with several years' worth of unopened *BMJs*. Behind his huge old desk was a small drawer, open, in which was an open copy of *Tristram Shandy*. There was a huge crush at the crematorium. After the service an old man who I did not know came up to me and said 'You're a doctor too, I hear, bet you're not as good as your Dad. I'll tell you this, he listened to you, didn't examine you much [I had worked that out], but he listened, and then he knew. Never wrong, never'. Well, I have often been wrong, but I have tried to listen. The secret of being a good GP is intimately tied up with the ability to listen, but more than that it is the ability to synthesise what you are hearing, filter it through the medical sieve, and share your understanding with your patient. This does require a certain involvement, which can float close to voyeurism and is done better by those with a tendency to curious gossiping, but it must stop short of true friendship. It is a professional relationship imbued with an intimacy that is often frightening to younger doctors.

That said, most of the cards and letters I have received allude to a friendship and a true sense of loss on behalf of the patients and their families. This 'friendship' is very real and perhaps engenders trust, which is such a valuable asset in the healing art. Continuity of care, currently threatened from several developments in primary care, is obviously highly valued by many, but the reality is that there will be less of it, so how will doctors in the future make a difference? The solution has to be by consulting well. If you are not going to know a patient over a long time-scale, it is even more important to get to what matters to them quickly and efficiently. This does require time, always a problem, but initial consultations of less than say ten minutes for all but the simplest transactions will be very unhelpful, and strategies of seeing patients through an event over a series of consultations must be in place. The 'doc in a box' future is to be resisted for everyone's sake.

Going back to the broccoli, I met Hazel there last week. She is 70, plump and has suffered lifelong disabling anxiety, but coped because of a truly great and caring human being, her husband Ron. She greeted me emotionally and told me Ron had died suddenly while I was in hospital myself. She was just the tiniest bit reproachful as she hugged me and said, 'and where were you when I needed you . . . you would have made such a difference'. I told the checkout girl that I had hayfever.

Chapter 10

Trust me, I'm a doctor

I will let you into an embarrassing secret – I like old Westerns. One of my favourites is John Ford's *Stagecoach* but at least I am in good company there, as Orson Welles is said to have watched it over 100 times before making *Citizen Kane*. One of the beguiling aspects of the film is the behaviour of the doctor. We meet him, debt ridden, fleeing town and hopelessly addicted to whiskey. We learn that his addiction may be related to the unspeakable horrors he has witnessed during the Civil War, and that he has abandoned all pretence of professionalism and sobriety. He insinuates himself shamelessly with a mouse of a whiskey salesman, and as the stagecoach rolls along through Indian country, he drinks the poor man's wares. Then, of course, comes the dramatic twist: a young cavalry officer's wife goes into labour at a stage halt, and medical skills, as well as plenty of hot water, are called for. One of the subplots has the socially despised 'tart with a heart' having to act as midwife to the upper-class lady. The doctor dramatically sobers up, aided by plenty of hot coffee, and proceeds to perform the necessary medical duties through a difficult but successful birth. So far so clichéd, still good, nonetheless. It is the scene after the birth that is particularly revealing. In the dark corridor the prostitute pours out her problems to the doctor; should she go away with the handsome young Ringo? Played, of course, by John Wayne. Should she tell him 'the sort of girl she is'? Could the doctor stop him going to a showdown, where he will almost certainly be killed? The point about these questions and requests to the newly rehabilitated doctor is that none of them is remotely medical. He is bemused but kindly and does his best, but why does she ask him these deeply personal questions? It is because she trusts him, and she does that because he has just proved himself, despite all his past failings, worthy of that trust.

Now the nature of this column relates to training future GPs, and from the above example we could concentrate on how to train doctors to gain the trust of their patients; there is enough in that subject for at least a couple of books. However, it seems to me that the more important training issues are how to train GPs to cope with the trust they will engender whether they are trying or not, and how to use it as a force for good in their patients' lives. Young doctors are not used to being trusted, their superiors in the hospital pecking order seldom do, and for most their impression is of being tolerated and no more. Trust itself is not an unmixed blessing; it carries with it responsibilities and duties and these can become burdens. One coping strategy is to ignore the human connection and not allow the human need for emotional trust to impinge on the consulting process, to remain matter of fact and aloof. An even worse strategy is, of course, to abuse it, as Shipman did, with truly terrifying consequences. But many others have also abused it, even though to a lesser extent, and most are not known to the General Medical Council.

So the first and most obvious lesson is that trust without integrity is a dangerous commodity. This sounds simple enough, but what is integrity in a medical setting? Seductions and wheedling your way into wills are obvious enough, but what about the more complex issues, for example personal care versus the greater good? Mass immunisation is the most obvious topical example. Trust me, have the MMR vaccination, we must prevent the threatened measles epidemic, and the scientific evidence against it is rubbish. When I make this statement to my patient my integrity is total, I believe what I have said to be true, and some of my more trusting patients will follow my advice, but many won't. Why not? Don't they trust me? I suspect Cherie Blair doesn't.

A recent *British Medical Journal* explores some of these issues in depth, in fact the whole issue is devoted to the communication of risk.[1] As far as 21st-century Western humans are concerned, it seems the size of the risk, for example autism from MMR, does not necessarily relate to the controversy it causes. We are also irritatingly irrational and as parents often neglect much greater risks, such as road traffic accidents, but this irrational behaviour seems understandable if parents are seen as trying to protect their children within the current social milieu. The less trusting may doubt my integrity, many know I am paid to vaccinate so I cannot be seen as unbiased, and medical integrity is based on current knowledge, which can always be found wanting. Think of hormone replacement therapy; for years a drug firm led the feminist crusade to free one sex from the tyranny of its hormones, to give stronger bones, better sex, a healthier heart, longer life, etc. Er, well as it turns out that's not exactly true, but I believed it all for a decade and when I discussed it my integrity was total, albeit misplaced, and I was trusted.

Integrity and screening is an even nastier conundrum. Some of the early advocates of cervical screening deliberately exaggerated the benefits and played down the harms for the greater good, and doctors like myself played along with this deception because it was too difficult to swim against the tide. I am not proud of my integrity over that issue.

Anyway, to go back to the old *Stagecoach*-type doctoring, in my early days in practice I looked after a serially divorced histrionic lady with a case file fatter than a family Bible from hundreds of psychosomatic complaints. She started a new relationship with a truly genuine, sensitive and caring man. This relationship, as far as I was concerned, had disaster written all over it, especially for the male. One evening surgery he came to see me and asked me the totally non-medical question: Should he marry her? Every reflex in my body was saying 'no, no, a thousand times, no'. But professionalism triumphed, for once, and I let him discuss the pros and cons as he saw them, contributed no embargoed medical information, and watched him leave with a heavy heart, wishing I could have saved him from the torment his life was about to become. The marriage, as it turned out, has been an unmitigated success, the psychosomatic complaints dried up at once and they are still happily together after 25 years. I thank God for my integrity on that occasion, and that it saved me from what would have been a disastrous breach of trust, though I would never have known and might even have felt quite smug at saving what I saw as a poor wretch from marital misery.

Another thought. How do we help our registrars with the trust of the dying? I have been lucky to be part of a practice in a town with a community hospital and have overseen the deaths of many patients. Because of this experience my palliative care skills are better than average and, partly because my practice is in the grounds of the hospital, frequent visiting has been easy. It is a real privilege to care for a fellow human being during a final irreversible illness; here their trust can be spoken or unspoken but is usually unmistakably etched in the eyes. A recent *British Medical Journal* article suggested that 'advance directives', or living wills, are pretty useless because the carers interpret them in the way their values and inclinations take them, but a good GP, with the trust of their patient, should know their wishes.[2] This can be a burden, as a painless speedy end in a hopeless situation is a common human wish, and not always easy to deliver in a society fearful of the slippery slope towards euthanasia. It is also often hard to gauge that moment when hope for recovery tips over into the realisation of dying. For some lucky ones this never happens, but for most the eyes dull and there is the pleading look full of realisation and, most heartfelt, sometimes of reproach. The look says, 'I trusted you, now help me'. I watched this transition in my wife, Sandra, who had been in the community hospital for several weeks with a terminal illness. My son saw it as well, but we were impotent to help other than to be there. Her GP saw it too and accepted the burden of trust, spoke to her, increased her sedation and she died peacefully without the reproach in the eye. In this case, of course, I was a relative, not a doctor and my trust in the GP and the nurses was total and not misplaced. But many young doctors shy away from the dying, uncertain of what they can contribute and afraid of the burden that is already on their shoulders. Their training must cover this area. We must give them the interpersonal and medical skills to be able to deliver on a contract they may not be aware that they have already signed up to.

References

1   *British Medical Journal* (2003) **327**(7417).
2   Thompson T, Barbour R and Schwartz L (2003) Adherence to advance directives in critical care decision making: vignette study. *British Medical Journal.* **327**: 1011.

Chapter 11

Modern general practice and the laboratory

What most GPs know about pathologists could be written in large capitals on their thumbnails. That is unless they happen to marry one, which is unlikely, as they never meet them. What most GPs know about modern pathology could probably be written in slightly smaller capitals. There are several reasons for this less than ideal state of affairs. Older GPs' memory of ancient lectures and unreadable textbooks has decayed with the passage of the years, and although they have been on many refresher courses, pathology per se has never been a strong draw: 'Let's go to the lecture on cardiology or diabetes – there will be passing mention of some of the latest clever tests, but more importantly this will tell us how to get the points for the NSFs and our new contract.' Everyone knows what points mean. They mean prizes or, more accurately, 'quality' money in the chronic disease management allowances. So to take diabetes and the laboratory as an example using the current version of the 'new' contract, a total of 99 points are up for grabs. Of those relating to the laboratory, 3 points are available for having a record of HbA_{1c} in the previous 15 months, and 11 points are available for practices that can achieve an HbA_{1c} of 10 or less in at least 85% of patients on their diabetic register in the last 15 months. There is a sliding scale of points from 85% to a threshold of 25%. If your brain is beginning to hurt, you are not alone, and this is but a tiny fraction of the Byzantine system that is being introduced. But let us press on. There are 16 points available if 50% of diabetics have an HbA_{1c} of 7.4 or less. Some committee in its wisdom, perhaps even with real live pathologists sitting on it, has decided that 7.4 is the magic figure, although there is a slightly worrying proviso that says 'or equivalent test/reference range depending on local laboratory.' This seems to provide a real opportunity for GPs and pathologists to get together to provide a perhaps more realistic target locally. Flattery and naked bribery seem to be the best tactics. If 90% of diabetic patients have had their serum creatinine levels measured in the last 15 months, that is another 3 points, and the same points apply to a measure of total cholesterol. Six points are available if 60% of diabetic patients have a serum cholesterol level of less than 5 mmol/l. It is worth noting that a detailed lipid profile, although much more useful, attracts no more points, so if you are just in it for the money such requests might decrease, which may even be a relief to an overworked laboratory. I, like many others, am unsure of the exact sums of money attached to these points, but for a superhuman practice (or one with a clever creative accounting system) the maximum number of points relating to the laboratory for diabetes would be 42, and a figure of £3,500 per average practice would not be too far away. Now in this brave new world of quality points, 70 points are available for distributing a patient survey, reflecting on it, chatting to the primary care trust and demonstrating a little bit of change. This will pull in £5,250 in the first year and £8,400 subsequently, and there are organisations which charge a fee of £60 that will do most of this for you. I write books on doctor–patient communication and am in favour of patient involvement, but it does seem that the points distribution could be construed as a little skewed.

In fact the whole ethos of measuring 'quality' in this target-driven way may have undesirable effects, not least on the very nature of the general practitioner and their relationship with the public. Targets encourage protocol-driven consulting, and there is a considerable risk that the patient's actual agenda – what really matters to them – will be subsumed in a checklist approach with an underlying whiff of medical totalitarianism. If this really does improve patient outcomes then the benefit may outweigh the harm, but the evidence on patient adherence/concordance with medical advice in chronic conditions is salutary and dispiriting. Moreover, there is some (albeit limited) evidence that more effective patient-centred consulting will improve adherence, although this style of consulting could easily be squeezed out of the repertoire.

Now to the future GP. The 12-point SHO rating scale from the JCPTGP (if you don't know, don't ask) dated August 2003, incorporating the GMC's *Good Medical Practice*, has as 1b 'Investigations.' This is part of 'an evolving portfolio' of personal and professional development of the young SHOs who have general practice as their career goal. In each six-month post they will be reviewed in the first two weeks, at three months and in the last two weeks. At each review there will be a 12-point rating scale, so back to 1b, which is in fact number 3. A total of 9 marks are available, with top marks for 'arranges, completes and acts on investigations intelligently, economically and diligently.' At the other end of the scale is 'inappropriate, random, unnecessary investigations, no thought given. Often fails to perform investigations requested', which to the mind of a slightly cynical GP sounds like the average outpatient clinic. This is then translated into a RITA, which can be satisfactory, satisfactory with minor concerns or unsatisfactory. Of course the matter of who does the assessment is key here, as is the 'diligence' of the process. This is likely to be extremely variable, but at least the intentions are good. And so into the GP registrar year and the Structured Trainer's Report. Specific clinical skill number 11 is obtaining venous access, or 'getting blood' in old speak. The only other mention relating to laboratory use is clinical judgement skill number 23 – 'the doctor undertakes appropriate examination (including investigations)' (their parentheses, not mine). There are 35 checkpoints in total.

Wearing another hat, I am Convenor of the MRCGP examining panel, and we have recently produced a detailed syllabus, available on the RCGP website, that is structured around but more detailed than *Good Medical Practice*. Doctors sitting the examination will have their knowledge of investigative pathology tested reliably by a comprehensive multiple-choice paper, their decision making explored in the oral examination and their overall consulting skills examined by submitting seven actual consultations on videotape. We are currently exploring methodologies for reliably examining both basic and complex clinical skills, including use of the laboratory. The advantage of including this in an examination is as an educational driver as well as an actual measure of the educational journey so far. The proposed curriculum for general practice is still under development, and I hope that practising pathologists will contribute to this debate and thus influence the future generalists and steer them towards knowledgeable use of finite laboratory resources.

Of course the real trouble with knowledge is that it keeps changing, and pathological tests are not immune from this. It is also clear that our evidence base is wafer thin in most instances and that tests, like the Bible, are capable of interpretation in many different ways. This should require practising clinicians to seek interpretation of meaning from those who might know more, namely clinical pathologists. I have to say that my experience of urgent advice from the duty pathologist over the phone has been excellent, but for the more day-to-day niggle it is hard to justify a phone call to an already over-committed NHS lackey. You know the sort of query – could HRT help this chap who was found to have low testosterone during screening after a hip fracture? Now is this a question for a pathologist or an endocrinologist? Perhaps there is scope for a sort of

'Pathologists R Us' interactive website with the usual FAQs and suggestions on whom to ask what and when.

The truth is that medicine and particularly primary care has been at a crossroads for some time, representing the collision of the art, the science, the workload, the money and the Government. I noticed in a survey of pathologists in the *ACP News* of summer 2003 that top of the list of reasons for liking pathology was the fact that there was no on call. Doughnuts featured surprisingly low on this list, as did 'not being in the department.' A GP survey would produce very similar results, although if my practice is any kind of guide, doughnuts would feature more prominently. The problem is, of course, who is going to do the on call. As the new contract steamrollers on, minor problems like this are ignored, as are those inherently difficult areas relating to screening, where pathologists and GPs nearly touch. The difficulty is the consent issue, cervical screening being a classic case. This article could turn into a tirade against the Machiavellian deception that has been at the core of such major and labour-intensive screening programmes, but it would do no good. Suffice to say this is an area where GPs and pathologists should get together and practise honesty and communication, with the intention that our patients be genuinely informed of the risks and benefits of these endeavours that are so lucrative to the GP and possibly to the pathologist.

Perhaps I could finish with two poems to illustrate the dilemma faced by the new GP. The first is the 1930s model espoused by the great WH Auden and the second is Marie Campkin's chilling modern version. What sort of GP do pathologists want?

Give me a doctor partridge plump,
short in the leg and broad in the rump,
an endomorph with gentle hands,
who'll never make absurd demands
that I abandon all my vices,
or pull a long face in a crisis,
but with a twinkle in his eye,
will tell me that I have to die.

Give me a doctor underweight,
computerised and up to date.
A businessman who understands
accountancy and target bands.

Who demonstrates sincere devotion
to audit and to health promotion –
but when my outlook's for the worse
refers me to the practice nurse.

Chapter 12

This is a fine mess you have gotten me into

My daughter is about to qualify as a doctor. My fatherly pride is enhanced by the knowledge that after six years (she took an intercalated BSc) she might at last pay her own mobile phone bill. She doesn't yet know which area of medicine she is going to concentrate on, but she seems 'medically' inclined; though she quite liked psychiatry, and does not rule out general practice, perhaps only to keep her dad happy. She will be the last of the old guard, the pre-PMETB generation, an unmodernised medical career so no new curriculum for her; well, maybe. Now, if she delayed qualification for a year by failing finals say (perish the thought), she would enter the brave new world of restructured training, continuous formative assessments, workplace-based assessments and as yet undefined summative assessments. Her pre-registration year will metamorphose into two foundation years, though as I write this there is no agreed structure, particularly to the second of these years, it just seems like a good idea. Whose?

If she wishes to be a physician, there are rumours that there will be an agreed general training, post-foundation, of four years; this will be a considerably streamlined version of the current system, plus an extra few years, depending on the complexity of the sub-specialty. Now what if she had been surgically inclined? I hear the current view is for a six-year training course, preferably snaffling year two of the foundation year. Again there will be extra years, depending on the complexity of the job, such as complex heart surgery, etc. A leading article in a recent *British Medical Journal* bemoaned the fact that more and more reforms resulted in less and less time for training. Before the Calman reforms and the impending Joint European Working Time Directive, the average number of hours spent in training for surgery was 30 000 hours; the Chief Medical Officer proposes to reduce this to 6000 hours. To quote the leading article: 'To become a competent surgeon in one fifth of the time once needed either requires genius, intensive practice, or lower standards. We are not geniuses.' Teaching intensity has not increased and training needs are often incompatible with a system geared increasingly to provide service not training. To quote this article again: 'Those of us lucky enough to be underway with our training on good teaching rotations can only feel relief that we are not in the cohort coming behind.' The details of the forth-coming reforms are not agreed yet, but it does seem clear that in most instances specialist training will be very significantly shortened.

This is all based on the competency theory: learn and demonstrate you have learned the appropriate competencies; when you have learned all the important ones then you are trained. If the full competency model is to be followed, time becomes irrelevant, but hospitals need structures and someone to actually do the work, so this is not very easy to actually implement. The trouble is that competency is all very well but it is not performance. Putting all the eggs in the competency basket may just produce a lot of scrambled egg rather than the omelette intended. Lower standards seem inevitable; even now a recent poll of consultant surgeons showed that two-thirds would not wish to be operated on by a Calman-trained consultant colleague.

OK, let's get to the meat. What about general practice? This, to share an oft-repeated phrase, is a time of opportunity and threat. As I write, it appears that the argument has been won to retain three years' GP training on top of the two foundation years. This is exciting, but whether the future product of such training schemes will be improved will of course depend on how useful the second foundation year turns out to be, as well as the quality of the three training years. Up to now most GP training has been a form of remedial teaching, undoing the bad habits and distorted values picked up between the latter years in medical school, the hospital experience and starting in supervised GP practice. If the second foundation year can undo some of this insidious harm it will be all well and good, but don't hold your breath. General-ism is still belittled in medical schools (personal communication from my daughter) and students do not rate it highly in the intellectual point-scoring stakes, though will often drift into it because the structure increasingly suits family life. The expressed wish to be GPs in most medical schools is now mostly below 20% and in some medical schools it is in single figures. This could be the sign of a dying vocation. Workforce planning for 2015 estimates there will be 60 000 consultants and 40 000 GPs; if this were a game, specialism clearly won the 20th century and is set to clear up in the 21st.

The lynchpin of the new GP training schemes will apparently be selection, though how this will actually work is a mystery to me. If the number of graduates actually wanting to do the job is falling and the number needed to train is actually rising, even my maths can work out that there will not exactly be a vast pool of punters to select from. So the sophisticated selection methods being developed in Sheffield and other places are all well and good, but in other hard-pressed deaneries the most important question in the selection process is likely to be: 'When can you start?' This is a situation many of us have been in before, but this time the rules are in the process of changing. There will be a curriculum; a well thought-out linked training programme; lots of work-based assessments; and a new endpoint, or possibly midpoint, assessment to replace the current MRCGP examination and summative assessment. One of my worries about this situation is related to the suggestion that if we select properly then our assessments will become less important because we will know we have already weeded out those who might currently fail summative assessment. But what if we don't select properly? Another worry is piloting; this will have to become live and be adjusted as the registrars are in post. Management of change has never up to now been a particular strength of the NHS and a clearer recipe for potential chaos may be hard to concoct. Now these arguments may seem a bit Luddite, there is no doubt that change is needed, but there is doubt about the sort of change needed to produce the optimum result for our patients, our young doctors and our medical teachers.

As an aside, you might like to take a pen and paper and work out the GP workforce implication for the next few years. Those graduating in 2004 (like my daughter) will finish GP vocational training in 2008 and perhaps take the last old-style MRCGP examination in that year. The 2005 graduate will take a year longer and be assessed by whatever new methodology has been agreed by then, but s/he will not complete the training until 2010. I wouldn't bother advertising for a partner in 2009, and the supply of handy locums is likely to be severely curtailed. I have a nasty feeling that when the politicians realise this there might be a drastic rethink. I hope I am wrong.

So after this fairly gloomy overview, do I have any brilliant suggestions? Well, in truth, not really, but I do know what is important. Experience is important, learning from it even more so, and that needs good intensive teaching and time to amass, to learn and to reflect. Communication is crucial, knowing is necessary but not sufficient, any future assessments must retain and preferably develop methodologies for testing the effectiveness of communication not just with patients, central though that is, but with colleagues, team members and outside organisations.

Competence will remain important to test at staging posts in the training, but we must not lose sight of the fact that it is performance that actually matters.

We generalists must fight back, we are not the failures who fell off Lord Moran's ladder and we do perform a complex, subtle, necessary and cost-effective job. It is very hard to learn how to effectively know a reasonable amount about an awful lot, which is the nature of generalism. It may be a lot easier in many cases to learn a lot about a little, which can be the nature of many specialties, yet it is the specialist who has the kudos and the generalist who is seen as slightly second rate. This is wrong, but this view has prevailed for more than a century. It must not prevail for a second century. We must grab the chance to enthuse, motivate and evangelise potential GPs and to create an education system worthy of high-quality, flexible doctors who can see patients as people and can tailor the medical requirements to their individual needs. It may be too late to persuade my daughter that we can really do this. It certainly seems too late for most of her contemporary student colleagues, but we must reverse this trend soon by getting our young GPs to enthuse their students. The future of family medicine depends on reversing the trends or soon we will all be specialists. Is that what you want?

Chapter 13

The pursuit of happiness

So what is it all about then? This being a doctor and this training lark, what is the nub of it all? I am still working at the answer but thought I could share with you how far I had got. I am at an age when looking backwards tends to be more productive than peering into crystal balls. A recent very enjoyable reunion promised to enlighten me just a little on what I had been doing as a trainer all of these years. You see a group of my registrars/trainees took me out for meal at my favourite restaurant recently. Since becoming a trainer in 1976, I have been privileged to train 21 doctors, as well as an eight-year stint as a course organiser. More than half actually came and several others sent their regrets and regards. We moved round after each course so by the end of the evening I had had a chance to ask everyone what it was they remembered as the most significant training experience. All of them, in some form or other, said friendship, a feeling of being welcomed and most talked of a deeper understanding as to why patients behave the way they do. The more honest ones remembered the somewhat *ad hoc* planning and the distinct lack of a portfolio philosophy, but all mentioned one word that fills me with self indulgent pride, they talked of enthusiasm. Many went on to add that their training year was a very happy one. My last registrar sat with my trainee 1977 vintage and exclaimed that she was only three then! And at least they both had happy memories.

In 1776, 200 years before I became a trainer, Thomas Jefferson and other notable colonists penned the first draft of the American Constitution. It begins: 'We hold these truths to be self evident, that all men are created equal, that they are endowed by their creator with certain unalienable rights, that among these are life, liberty and the pursuit of happiness.' Now as doctors it is clearly our job to help with the right to life, though difficult issues like the abortion and *in vitro* fertilisation debates mean that the ethics of whose life can get difficult. As a profession our role in the right to liberty is not self evident, to me at least; and what is our role in the pursuit of happiness? Perhaps we should start with what the ingredients of happiness are; we could then concoct a recipe Delia style. Of course we all know it doesn't work that way; one man's happiness is his wife's misery, if we take football on the telly as an example. Maybe the founding fathers were near the mark, it is the pursuit that is the unalienable right, actually catching happiness is a rare event and it is such a phantasmagorical substance that it usually escapes through the net very quickly.

Happiness is a state of mind, and some are more prone to catch it than others, but it is a very rare human being who is never happy, and such an individual in our society's medical model would probably be considered ill. Now I am intrinsically an optimist, normally full of enthusiasm about this and that, as my registrars remember, and often, if I stop to think about it, find myself cheerful enough to class as happy in my internal lexicon. This is usually without any obvious pursuit of the ephemeral feeling. Those of you who have gamely followed this column for some time will be dimly aware that all was not well in Château Tate for some while, severe personal illness and acute on chronic deterioration leading to the untimely death of my wife. Work stopped, the future looked bleak, enthusiasm dried up as quickly as a puddle in the sunshine, and yes the previously ever nearby happiness evaporated too. Friends did their best, my children were heroic, and the doctors too tried very hard with my wife, at least allowing her a dignified death. My own doctors, the cardiologists and cardiac surgeons patched me up, and chivvied me for not getting better. For months everything was an effort, lifting an arm was like lifting 20 kg at the gym, the feeling of fatigue never lifted, and the future looked grey and uninviting. In my working life I have never been certain of the clear aetiological mix that makes up chronic fatigue conditions but I had never met anyone with those sorts of conditions who appeared happy, while on the contrary I regularly saw people with severe disability and even terminal illness who were extremely cheerful and apparently quite happy. This is not claiming a depressive causation, but a lack of happiness seemed part of the syndrome. The pursuit seemed also distorted, often that seemed to be a pursuit for recognition of suffering rather than for that elusive happiness. Looking inside myself I saw no pursuit of anything, just resignation and a sort of all-embracing flatness. Bereavement, major surgery and loss of job are of course all serious events, but aided by my son and daughter somehow a seed was sown that wallowing was not an option, and that I had quickly to learn how to restart the pursuit of the elusive. 'Carpe diem' as they say. Then I met someone who needed some happiness too, we liked each other's company instantly and the fatigue disappeared almost overnight. This all sounds a bit trite, like a prescription from a Ken Dodd song, but do we doctors think about happiness enough? And should we train for it?

The one other positive contribution I had made to my registrars' thinking related to why people do what they do, particularly of course in relation to illness behaviour. This comes down to an interest in the ubiquitous health belief – now I collect health beliefs like others collect stamps. A couple of favourites to illustrate the point: the lady who loved her 'Aquarius' cream for her psoriasis, 'it works because I am Gemini, and we are very influenced by Aquarius' she told me with not a trace of irony. Or the nuclear scientist who was convinced his intermittent atrial fibrillation was directly related to the amount and type of beer he drank and kept detailed graphs of the correlation, while not altering his drinking habits one jot, but turning up with the graphs in quadruple colours every month for inspection. On reflection, the most interesting health beliefs seem to relate to the pursuit of a goal that is perceived by the patient to lead to an increased chance of happiness. These health beliefs may be absolutely crucial to the understanding of illness behaviour. A patient of mine was a young diabetic mother with two teenage children. She was apparently very conscientious about looking after her diabetes, but her sugars fluctuated wildly as did her weight. She was initially adamant that she stuck rigidly to her diet. Over several consultations the truth gradually emerged and it was complex. Her marriage had failed; she was a single working mother with a high pressure job and a need to keep up appearances by looking attractive. She knew from her own experience that if her sugar was high for a period of time she would lose weight and, in her conviction, look more attractive and be more likely to find another partner and so be happier. But equally significant was her fear of long-term diabetic complications and her real need to keep her sugar levels within a reasonable range, and in her deep-rooted belief this meant that her weight must be controlled at all costs. This belief led to the absolutely paradoxical behaviour of secret chocolate binge eating, to raise the sugar and so lose weight; this was of course also a guiltily pleasurable foible, and to add to it allowed her to believe that such an irrational activity could in fact make her slim and attractive, and so increase her confidence and self-esteem which were directly linked to the achievement of her personal happiness. Only by dissection of these beliefs could she be helped to achieve satisfactory control and a weight she could accept. And how did I find this out? Well I picked up a few cues and followed them, I probed and used the knowledge gained about her social and psychological circum-stances and I searched out her deeply hidden (from health professionals) health beliefs; in the light of these beliefs we then negotiated a treatment and management plan and worked on a useful follow-up regime. Those of you who have registrars taking the Member of the Royal College of General Practitioners (MRCGP) video may recognise those behaviours. The word is that this exam is to go the way of all flesh, some of you will be pleased I know, but you will not be surprised to be told that I find that a deep sadness. Still that is another story and I am going back to the pursuit, the good news is that recently the catching net doesn't seem quite so full of holes.

Chapter 14

Managing the conflict in the consultation between data entry and caring

We GPs have a new contract; it is in the rhetoric quality driven. The ethos is characterised by the evidence-based mantra, and to old war horses like me it looks like a huge extension of the old item of service philosophy that has made our salaries such a Byzantine calculation for decades. I make the point about the relative lack of newness just to keep our feet on the ground, but the scale is unprecedented and the effect on day-to-day consulting profound. One problem is the nature of the new point scoring, and we all know what points mean, they mean prizes, and the incentive to win prizes is ingrained in every modern human, even including GPs and certainly including switched on practice managers. Prizes skew our behaviour, but for the better?

In fact the whole profession is aware that the prevailing ethos of measuring 'quality' in this target-driven way may have undesirable effects, not least on the very nature of GPs' relationship with the public. Targets encourage protocol-driven consultations, and there is a considerable risk of overlooking the patient's actual agenda, with what really matters to them being subsumed in a checklist approach – with an underlying whiff of medical totalitarianism. If this really does improve patient outcomes then the benefit may outweigh the harm, but the evidence on patient adherence and concordance with medical advice in chronic conditions is salutary and dispiriting. There is some, but limited, evidence that more effective patient-centred consulting will improve adherence, though this style of consulting could easily be squeezed out of the repertoire in a target-driven culture. Consumer surveys that appear on a weekly basis these days continually stress the public's wish for more information and mostly for more involvement in decisions taken that affect their own health.

The public has now cottoned on to at least some of the implications of this target-driven culture and this has done nothing for their trust in their GP's advice. The MMR and now the wider child immunisation debate has released a Pandora's Box of medieval superstitions mixed with pseudo-science, not all of this on the patient's side. The carefully built wall of trust has had a large hole blown in it, and the ensuing gale is threatening the very structure of the patient/healthcare relationship. Some of the conflict, for that is what it is, relates to the greater good argument. The population's health versus the individual's and the arguments, the per-spectives and the implications are quite different when viewed from the public health strategy room at the Department of Health and the worried parents overdosed on a diet of partially digested internetinfosludge and the high-calorie Daily Mailomania. The big question is of course, in this increasingly hysterical yet constrained climate is it still possible to do and to train for reasonable patient-centred best practice? The real conflict is between patient involvement, choice and achieving targets. Maybe every 85-year-old should take five tabs a day to keep their blood pressure and cholesterol down, but no annoying tests or doctor-induced interven-tions so that they can totter on until 90. The trouble is many of them would welcome a quick MI, but perhaps not a stroke. As a patient this would not be too onerous a strategy, and fulfils Kingsley Amis' dictum that no pleasure in life is worth forgoing for an extra four years in a nursing home in Weston-super-Mare. But if we don't immunise our children, then back come the diseases. Patients really don't like too much choice, all the worry over potential but rare side-effects cloud the issues; and the reality of life, that choices, options and facts are often brutal, is missed. If you don't like the potential side-effects, then would you rather have the disease – now you choose?

A recent study into the real feasibility of evidence-based choice as a model for the new general practice showed that many of us had major worries, such as the relative lack of evidence for most conditions and the extreme scarcity of evidence derived from the patient's perspective, and many felt that the whole effort was just too time-consuming. Perhaps assessing, interpreting and sharing evidence with our patients could have such an adverse impact on the limited time available for dealing with all the other aspects of patient care that the overall effect will be to reduce access to the service and so its effectiveness. That is not to denigrate the evidence-based medicine (EBM) bandwagon. The appropriate use of good primary care-based research evidence must be encouraged, but the incentives to go down this road need tempering or both our patient's

autonomy and the fair distribution of finite resources will be compro-
mised.[1]

So how are we going to train our new generation of doctors to surmount
these dilemmas? Is it possible to care and use a computer properly in the
consulting room? I think the answer is yes, but it is skilful and needs
instruction and practice; so where do we start?

How about the environment of the encounter to get us started?
Consulting room layout is important, exactly how important research
has not entirely clarified, but it seems axiomatic that if both doctors and
patients want some form of sharing then the structure and the ambience
must facilitate that. Both parties should be able to see the screen, but
there is a caveat even here; in consultations where a third party is present
there is a real confidentiality issue. I once ruined my relationship with a
teenage girl when in her mother's presence I flicked to the screen to
prescribe some salbutamol and Mum saw the repeat pill script. The
ensuing open row was a salutary experience. This means that the
computer screen must be mobile and in third party consultations explicit
permission must be sought to display personal information visible to that
party. Sharing information using a computer screen is a powerful tool,
tends to improve recall and certainly improves evidence-based patient
choice.

There is then the question of timing. How long does the patient get to
express their agenda before the doctor takes over? In a diabetic clinic the
medical agenda will dominate, not always to the patient's benefit, and in
open surgery how long is it till the blood pressure is checked? If there is to
be a structured data-entering culture then is there still time to structure
the consultation to allow the impingement of our patient's experience,
their fears and desires, and to clarify what it is that they have come to us
about. The use of time is probably the most helpful skill GP trainers can
impart to their registrars. Having watched far more videos of young
doctors consulting than is good for one's health, I can categorically state
that the majority of young registrars halfway to three-quarters through
their year are not very skilful at time management. Their mentors can
usually achieve similar outcomes in a lot less time, and not necessarily at
the expense of what matters to the patient. This requires practice, like
learning the piano, and it requires gentle and expert feedback based on
structured observation of performance. Professional expertise is based on
the lessons learned from those day-to-day bread and butter encounters.
Many registrars see a lot of patients but appear not to have learned too
much from these exchanges. This has to be the fault of the trainer whose

job it is to chisel the beautiful sculpture of experience from the unpromising rock of a morning surgery.

Many of the really cutting-edge developments in consultation thinking and teaching relate to this transition from novice, to reasonable competence, to day-to-day proficiency, to expert. A lot of empirical evidence suggests that many, perhaps even most, never reach true expertise. And how would we define that expertise in the current climate that is so full of tensions between checklist necessities, NICE guidelines and true patient-centredness? Here is my definition, an expert modern consulter will at the start seek to find out what it is that matters to the patient, and this requires respect and communicative expertise. Clinical competence is an absolute necessity, as is a highly developed sense of pattern recognition. The ability to synthesise the clinical necessities with the communicative imperative to achieve a shared understanding and shared management plan will be well developed. The consulter will be able to deal with a wide range of challenges, be able to cope with the ever-present uncertainty and to respond to their intuition, yet remain focused and appropriate in the use of resources, which includes the use of time. Throughout this immensely skilful process our consulter must remain the patient's advocate. There you are, not much to ask for is it? Someone who can do all this on a day-to-day basis is a valuable member of our society and deserves recognition and reward. So we must fight for this sort of consulter to be recognised and we must denigrate the purely checklist techniques that squeeze both the effectiveness and the humanity out of our surgeries.

Reference

1 Ford S, Schofield T and Hope T (2002) Barriers to the evidence-based patient choice (EBPC) consultation. *Patient Education & Counseling* 47: 179–85.

Chapter 15

To understand everything is to forgive everything?

My last registrar asked me not long before she left how I could remain so calm and apparently understanding with Barbara*, who was forever in the surgery and had the most complex and hair-raising repeat medication of opiates, antidepressives and anxiolytics. I set off on the explanation as to why Barbara had reached the state she was now in.

At time of our first meeting in 1974, Barbara was 26, attractive, vivacious, and married to an ambitious young accountant with prospects. She had one daughter, Shula, aged two, and was pregnant again. I supervised her normal pregnancy and even delivered her of Tom, a small noisy baby, via low cavity forceps for delay in the second stage; this was in the long-since defunct maternity unit in the local cottage hospital. Delivering babies, in some cases more than the act of procreating them, seems to produce a sort of bond between people. It was to be so with Barbara and me, but sadly Tom soon showed signs of heart problems. He failed to thrive, remained a slate bluey colour and the heart sounds were non-specifically abnormal. He was transferred to the local teaching hospital, and then for further investigation into a specialist unit in London. It slowly transpired that he had a severe congenital abnormality of the pulmonary artery, along with some other defects, and that his prospects for living past infancy were slim. Barbara and her husband were understandably hit very hard by this news and Barbara became depressed, which deepened over some weeks until she needed hospital admission without Tom or Shula, who were looked after by her husband's parents. She made a slow and shaky recovery. After her discharge I visited her at home several times, as was the norm then. She confided that she did not want to love Tom too deeply as the pain of his dying would then be too much to bear, and that she felt guilty about having these feelings. She was also guilt-ridden about neglecting her daughter and felt guilty too about

---

* Not her real name. Names and details have been changed to protect identities.

her lack of sexual feeling for her outwardly stolid but inwardly very distressed husband.

This situation never really resolved itself and the years went by, Tom did not die in infancy and by the age of five was a strong-willed, very intelligent little boy, fiercely angry at the constraints placed on him by his own body, and, as he saw it, his overprotective mother. His sister had retreated into a world of dolls and fantasy friends. Bill, the husband, kept getting promoted. Barbara was in a state of constant hyper-awareness of every breath Tom was taking, and constantly trailed the little lad round every specialist in the land, receiving many different opinions, but no help. She was convinced a heart transplant would be a solution, very reluctantly accepting that even this would not cure the anomaly buried deep in the lungs, that only a combined transplant would do, but at that time was not an option. Tom carried on living a disabled and fraught but very contributive existence. Wherever he spent time he made an impression, leaving his mark on carers, teachers, friends, doctors and indelibly on his family.

Seven more years passed, Tom had frequent collapses that threatened but did not lead to death; Barbara carried on searching, smoked constantly and developed a series of intractable symptoms too long to list. More and more doctors became involved, and care became increasingly fragmented. I hardly ever saw Bill, who was now a senior partner in a large firm, and Shula was becoming an increasingly withdrawn and sullen teenager. When Tom's valiant heart began to finally fail, both parents wanted him at home. His final illness lasted a week and I visited two to three times a day, which was made easier as they lived near the surgery. With advice we gave him sedation to ease his obvious suffering, but Barbara nursed him constantly, cleaning him, giving him drinks, always trying to comfort him. At breakfast time one morning while I was visiting, Tom sat up, stared into his mother's eyes only a few inches away, and screamed at her, 'I hate you, I hate you', and fell back dead. There are silences and silences, this was the second sort. Bill pulled Tom's lifeless body to his chest and sobbed convulsively; Barbara didn't move and stared out of the window. I couldn't trust myself to speak and was effectively useless, just able to touch Barbara on the shoulder in a pathetic gesture of sharing her pain. A minute or an hour went by, and then the room filled with a slow moan, starting soft and melancholic, building over eons to a screaming high-pitched wail of such intensity and pain that I can hear it now. It had not been easy initially to localise the sound to an individual but by now Barbara's head was thrown back and she was shaking both Bill and the departed Tom. The sound wouldn't stop, perhaps it still hasn't.

Weeks later Barbara confessed to me that Tom was haunting her. Standing by her bed rotting and accusing her with hate-filled eyes. My psychiatrist friend had name for it, but the image haunted me too. Gallons of platitudes were poured on Tom's unkind death, bucketloads of 'you did your best, you have nothing to reproach yourself for' type remarks, streams of 'you know he didn't mean it', but Barbara drowned in her river of grief. Bill was nearly swept away and Shula tried to cling onto the bank, but the supporting branch that had been her parents had broken, so she went downstream too. She literally lost herself in a 'bad crowd', became hooked on heroin, and spent some time in a young offenders unit.

Barbara's drowning was by extreme illness behaviour. Freud would have termed it hysterical conversion, a more modern but ugly word would describe it as somatisation. It seemed that Barbara's overwhelmed coping mechanisms tried in the last resort to fight fire with fire, or in her case pain with pain. She started the round of specialists again, low back pain and pain in the kidney regions being the main symptoms. Several esoteric diagnoses appeared, some seemingly dependent on the amount of money changing hands. The private medical subscription was soon enormous. Various strategies were adopted and drugs were added to her cocktail on a seemingly random haphazard basis. None of them worked but they became needed and the need escalated; paracetamol became dihydrocodeine, became morphine and finally heroin. Anxiolytics went from diazepam 2–5–10 to lorazepam, etc., and the same with antidepressants. Ten years after Tom's death, mother and daughter were both addicted to heroin, by differing routes, and Bill was still doing his best to cope, but thinking of early retirement. More than ten doctors and at least ten other professionals were involved with Barbara, but who was in charge? Balint's famous collusion of anonymity was being starkly illustrated. I tried, honestly I did, and a few times we managed meetings of Barbara, Bill, myself, the pain relief specialist, the psychiatrist and the cognitive therapist. We adopted strategies, created rules that were always broken but always for understandable reasons. The partners got more and more upset if I was away at having to provide repeat prescriptions for regimes that they were profoundly uncomfortable with. Barbara, conscious of this pressure, over-ordered lest she ran out, but in so doing increased her consumption, fuelling the addiction, increasing the pressure and magnifying the disapproval.

It was at about this stage that my registrar asked me how I could remain so outwardly calm about this pressure for drugs, therapy, care and attention that seemed all but insatiable. The truth is the calm was the outward manifestation of an inner guilt. It is all very well to say that if you know everything then you will forgive everything, this phrase sounds much better in French by the way, but forgiving isn't solving. I was guilty that my understanding and my forgiveness, however hard won, had not actually been enough to prevent the life-destroying medicalisation of a human being I genuinely cared for. I wasn't the only healthcare professional who had failed, but I was the lynchpin, the co-ordinator, and to assuage my guilt I acquiesced to most of Barbara's requests. My partners understandably thought this was taking a profoundly unhelpful easy option, and objectively they were right, but at the emotional level I wanted to make amends for Tom's death and my own inability to help relieve her suffering. Over the years this frustration even came out as anger, the glacial calm sometimes being replaced by petulant frustration surrounding repeat prescription requests. It has long been known that many long-term repeats represent a truce situation between doctor and patient, and this was always an uneasy truce, releasing painful emotions on both sides when the status quo was disturbed. I eventually let my registrar see a glimpse of the real, frustrated and not calm me. I suspect neither she nor I found this revelation particularly edifying.

So is there an end to this story? Well, not really, but Shula is off drugs, Bill has retired and seems happier than for ages, Barbara is still damaged but undoubtedly better and now adhering to a strict regime prescribed outwith the practice by the local addiction unit, and I have retired too, breaking the continuity, the dependence and so helping Barbara to improve. They all sent me a lovely retirement card. Doctors who know and forgive may still not improve your health, and continuity may not always be for the best, but it usually is.

Chapter 16

Depression: another disease of our time

NICE has spoken. We are overusing antidepressants, GPs should only use them 'when appropriate' and there should be more cognitive behaviour therapy, though quite where all the therapists will come from is unclear. There are lots of 'counsellors' but not that many really good ones, in my own experience. Those of us who have been GPs for more than a decade will clearly remember the 'defeat depression' campaign inspired by the notion promulgated by the psychiatrists that GPs were prescribing too few anti-depressants, and therefore clearly under-diagnosing such a debilitating and potentially serious condition. Have we now improved too much? While you are pondering that one I will ask you another couple of questions. What is depression and what is the threshold for prescribing drugs?

The late and greatly missed Roy Porter, in his chapter on Mental Illness in the *Cambridge Illustrated History of Medicine*, concludes by saying 'there is little agreement as to what mental illness truly is'.[1] In the 1970s, Thomas Szasz wrote: 'psychiatry is conventionally defined as a medical speciality [sic] concerned with the diagnosis and treatment of mental diseases. I submit that this definition, which is still widely accepted, places psychiatry in the company of alchemy and astrology and commits it to the category of pseudoscience. The reason for this is that there is no such thing as "mental illness"'.[2]

I was in Vienna recently and visited the museum of the most influential psychiatrist ever, Sigmund Freud. To be honest he has never been a hero of mine, and my assessment is that he contributed more than his fair share to the development of the introspective, self-indulgent society we have become. A clever, brave, irascible and eternally curious man, he spent the latter years of his life trying to prove that the iconoclastic Pharaoh Akhenaton was in fact the biblical Moses. He may have been right about that, but he certainly was not right about the interpretation of dreams or the mumbo-jumbo that became the religion of psychoanalysis.

During my visit the inner sanctum was filled by a large group of mainly young women who would not be moved on. Their eyes shone, they exuded excitement and awe; it was if they were in the presence of a deity, and there was not a shadow of a doubt that they 'believed' in Freud at that moment. Belief is part of our problem with depression; psychiatrists have chiselled out a syndrome with clear markers and definitions. This is now widely accepted by our society, who now firmly believe in depression, and GPs, who are part of society, are the faithful disciples who diagnose it day in and day out, whether too much, too little or about right depends on your viewpoint.

Shellshock, which has slowly metamorphosed into post-traumatic stress disorder (PTSD), is an interesting comparison; Pat Barker's wonderful *Ghost Road* trilogy reminds us of the absolutely brutal treatment of this condition during and after the First World War.[3] At that time society and psychiatrists did not really accept a severe stress reaction related to horrific experiences; there was an underlying feeling of incipient cowardice laced with a certain lack of moral fibre. This allowed a small band of 'physical psychiatrists' to effectively torture patients out of their symptoms, and the success rate was very high. Nowadays depression is accepted as a legitimate reason for killing oneself, for having long periods off work, for retiring early, for not looking after oneself or others and, perhaps most importantly, it is a gold-plated admission to the 'sick role'. You may have detected a whiff of cynicism on my part, but in reality I am just as confused as you are. There are many people who appear depressed by the criteria we currently accept who get better if they take the tablets prescribed by me, irrespective of apparent causation or lack of it, and are grateful for my ministrations. There are others who don't, but who are helped by other methodologies, from the still mysterious electroconvulsive therapy (ECT), to cognitive behaviour therapy (CBT), to group and family therapy, to one-to-one structured or unstructured counselling, etc.

When I was a ship's surgeon, more than 30 years ago, the ex-RN dispenser who treated the crew had a three-stage treatment for depression; stage 4 was to see me. It went like this:

1 'Pull yourself together and here is a bottle of red medicine.'
2 'Not you again, bl**dy get out more and here is the stronger green medicine.'
3 'Right! This time it's the Black Draught for you. Take it twice a day and I don't want to see you back.'

The Black Draught was liquid senna, and I never saw a case of depression. The culture on the ship was not conducive for the illness. Of course, many famous people have suffered depressive episodes. Two that come to mind are Winston Churchill, who had the family 'black dog', and Spike Milligan, who was famous for his manic depression. Both, however, led startlingly successful lives. The involutional melancholia of the Victorians was recognisably similar to the modern syndrome, and in the century before that Dr Johnson remarked: 'Melancholy, indeed, should be diverted by every means but drinking'. To my own chagrin, I went through a short phase myself, hated the loss of control over my mood and was mightily relieved when one day it just went, without treatment. So I repeat, what is it? And when should I prescribe for it?

You have already gathered that I don't know the answer to those questions, though as a 30-year coalface GP I do have a feel for it. As with breeds of dog, I like to think I can recognise it when it matters and treat it effectively too. And what about our registrars? Well, I can help there, having just watched over 70 registrars deal with the same simulation of the depressed young man. One great advantage of simulation over real life is that we know the script. In this script the patient is non-specifically depressed, has financial worries, which may be causal, some marital worries, which may be effect, he is sleeping badly, with characteristic early waking, and drinking too much. He has one hobby, shooting, and he owns his own guns. His scripted opening gambit is to ask for something to help him sleep and to look gloomy; he has thought of suicide but does not think he ever really will do it.

As you will understand, the young doctors' performances varied greatly, but some behaviours were into the 90% level. They were: drug prescribing (100%, NICE please note), referral to counselling, and an explanation of the illness depression. Around 80% made some attempt to involve the patient in their own treatment. So far so good (or bad if you are from NICE), but other more worrying behaviours were also in the 90% level. Alcohol was almost never discussed seriously, only two got to the shotguns, and neither made a real issue of it, although some sort of suicide assessment was present in about 70% of encounters. There was a lot of 'you have what we doctors call depression' and an overwhelming belief in counselling, though less than 10% mentioned CBT specifically as the only validated form. The drug prescribing was also fascinating. Amitriptyline had its advocates and fluoxetine was the second most popular, but way out in front was citalopram. Of course, NICE recognises that our drug firms have a deeply vested interest in prescribing for depression, to the extent of covering up unhelpful results in various trials. It is in the drug firm's interest to maintain a common, easily recognised condition that will be helped by specifically designed drugs. Our young doctors have clearly bought into this philosophy. Simulation may also stifle natural consulting ability, and in fact may only be measuring the ability to act. This did seem to be true for a few, and could explain the other major behaviour that was conspicuously lacking: curiosity. Over 90% of the young doctors knew no more about that young man as a human being by the end of the consultation; perhaps empathy is difficult to simulate. There is also the time pressure of ten minutes imposed by the constraints of the simulation, which may discourage any deeper exploration. But what was clear was that 100% of new doctors saw a depressed mood as a cause for medical intervention, and that intervention was primarily pharmacological.

Those enthusiasts who initiated the 'defeat depression' campaign must be gratified, though management of suicidal risk seems very superficial if the simulation is any guide. Recent figures, however, seem to indicate a fairly dramatic fall in the national suicide rate in the last decade. Could this be due to early therapy or just changes in the national mood? The underlying current in my mind is just how useful is this societal medicalisation of mood? The oft-asked question is 'Where does unhappiness stop and depression begin?' and the recent massive tsunami can help us focus on the answer. In the outpouring of aid for Sri Lanka, Indonesia, Southern India and Thailand, will there be crates of citalopram as well as bus loads of counsellors? And if there are, how much good will they do? We do know now that in many cases so-called counselling in disaster situations does more harm than good, which leads one to further suggest that the 'depressification' of human distress, misery, mourning and frustrated goals is an inherently bad adaptive strategy and only tolerable in a society that can allow itself that luxury.

References

1 Porter R (ed) (1996) *The Cambridge Illustrated History of Medicine*. Cambridge University Press: Cambridge.
2 Szasz TS (1972) *The Myth of Mental Illness: foundations of a theory of personal conduct*. Granada: London.
3 Barker P (2004) *Ghost Road*. Penguin: London.

Chapter 17

What is the secret of healing?

I know the answer to this question and it is walnuts, but you will have to read the rest of these musings to find out why. There was a motion put forward to a recent RCGP council meeting to the effect that the College should take more cognisance of complementary medicine with the implication that some standard setting would not go amiss. In the subsequent debate there were warnings of fearsome and little-known interactions between Granny's Ginkgo and her warfarin, of the risk of paraplegia from having one's neck cricked by a manipulator of some tribe or other, and an overwhelming feeling of incipient quackery mixed with annoying pseudo-science, especially annoying because at least half of our patients use some form of alternative medicine, usually without telling us. How can they be so gullible! There was then a contribution pointing out the dangers of modern medicine, citing the recent CoX2 debacle, where at least two mainstream flashy new arthritic wonder drugs have killed more people in a couple of years than *Ginkgo biloba* has done in its entire usage, pointing out that the evidence base for physiotherapy is no better than for osteopathy and probably worse than for chiropractic and that many common surgical procedures have a wafer-thin evidence base. Others tried to produce a hierarchy with acupuncture and chiropractic at the top and reflexology at the bottom, but this attempted ordering of the essentially random seemed doomed to failure. Council squared the circle by appointing a working party and hurriedly moving on, but all of us are firmly caught up in this debate, which is in essence about the nature of healing.

Our patients' expectations related to medicine's ability to cure continues to grow exponentially while our ability to treat much of most minor ailments is probably decreasing. Take common childhood illness, for example. When I started in practice over 30 years ago there was more in the GP's armament than now. There was aspirin, far more effective than paracetamol for hot miserable children; there were real antispasmodics for colic, gripe water that could get you banned from driving, sedatives that sedated children and cough mixtures you could stand your spoon up in. These have all gone, rightly or wrongly. We are left with paracetamol and dilute ibuprofen only; antibiotics are now so frowned on that a huge sense of guilt arises in every GP's psyche each time they are prescribed.

The resultant communication between doctor and anxious parent is now seriously flawed. It can be illuminating using the old ideas, concerns and expectations model. Take the anxious young mother to start with.

Her ideas: My child is unwell; he needs urgently checking by a doctor. He is distressed and in pain and these need relieving as quickly as possible. I think he has an ear infection because he is pulling them a lot.

Her concerns: My child might be seriously ill, could it be meningitis? She is concerned too that the doctor might not take her worries seriously and will make a mistake about the severity of the illness. She is worried that she won't know the doctor as there seems to be a different one every time she goes, and some talk in a medical language that she doesn't understand but doesn't like to admit to.

Her expectations: These are clouded by her worries, but include the idea of a curative prescription, the possibility of a hospital admission and the difficulties of getting to, seeing and understanding doctors.

Now take the doctor's understanding.

My ideas: This child is the fifth hot, cross under one-year-old I have seen today. What does mum expect of me? This is a self-limiting illness caused by a germ whose name I don't know, but as most infections just get better the likelihood is that this one will too.

My concerns: This mum is distressed and angry, is it just because of the illness? Is the child really ill? How much reassurance can I give?

My expectations: Mum will want antibiotics but I must educate her not to expect them for all childhood illnesses. If I get it wrong she may call out the creaking night service later tonight.

The consultation starts badly because of Mum's difficulty getting to see me: 'I haven't seen you for so long I thought you had retired'. I go on the defensive but try to soothe things by examining the cross child thoroughly. This reveals nothing except pink drums probably caused by screaming and a temperature of 39°C. The stark truth is that other than reassurance I have nothing to offer. Mum may interpret this as bloody-mindedness or professional negligence, a wilful withholding of cure and protection that her distressed child so manifestly needs. I may crack, providing the amoxicillin, perpetuating the saga.

Research from Little *et al.* at Southampton suggests that ascertaining and coping with Mum's concerns is the most effective way of dealing with such consultations, but that for many the only way to do that is by antibiotic prescribing.[1] So what do we modern doctors do? We have antibiotics that don't work but which parents want and we have lost our old weapons, placebos and magic. We still have caritas, but sometimes our patients don't believe that. The science has replaced the art and in so doing has lessened our ability to treat and manage minor illness. We must not forget, however, that we are pretty good and getting better at the bigger stuff. Cancer treatment, especially haematological, has improved dramatically, though our progress on the solid tumour front is still disappointing. Heart surgery is a miracle, a fact I can personally testify to. Joint surgery, hips and knees especially, has revolutionised so many lives. Medical treatment for diabetes, asthma and most of the infectious diseases has changed our world, and given millions worthwhile lives that they would not have had otherwise, and in all of these areas complementary or alternative medicine offers little except false hope and occasional wilful negligence that prevents conventional cure.

So here is the healing dilemma: why is modern medicine so relatively good at the big stuff and so ineffective in the minor illness domain? This debate concerns us GPs more than our specialist colleagues who are in most cases a lot clearer about what it is they are doing to heal those referred to them. They are protected by their scientific fort, their wall of evidence-based medicine (EBM), and their stockade of randomised controlled trials. Now we know that this stockade is often as flimsy as the one Davey Crockett defended with his 20 or so Tennesseans against Santa Anna's army at the Alamo, and we all know what happened there, but they did at least hold out for a while, and the other rebels went on to win. To carry on the warlike analogy, are we GPs caught out in the open or are we the ones who are going to win in the end?

Historically, doctors have never been so effective. There is evidence that the Roman Legion surgeons were pretty good at what they did, but still not in the same league as modern medicine. For most of the last two thousand years, doctors were more likely to dispose of you in a variety of painful and undignified ways than to actually heal you. The Age of Enlightenment coincided with the Age of Heroic Medicine, a time of bleeding and purging to the brink of death and often past it. This was not a healing era, yet the era we are living in really is. I think the main problem we generalists are now facing is certainty, or the lack of it. Doctors and patients both really dislike uncertainty, it is the biggest problem our registrars face on entering general practice, and then trendy trainers like me make it worse by advising a sharing approach. Sharing what? Well, uncertainty, of course. This is where our complementary colleagues have the edge, they eliminate uncertainty; there is always an explanation for why the therapy didn't work. You know the baked bean strategy, don't you? 'Well, my dear, I am sorry your baked beans didn't cure your headache, perhaps you took too many, or maybe the wrong sort. Shall we try the Amazonian ones this time? Or of course, perhaps you took too few, we should double the dose. Etc.' Now we doctors have been known to dabble in this strategy too, but we are nowhere near as good at it, probably because in our heart of hearts we don't really believe.

At last we near the truth; let me tell you of an old GP colleague who drove a Rolls Royce and had a huge private practice. This was 30 years ago, I hasten to add. He dabbled in many therapies, but was particularly fond of manipulation. Being a huge man, 6ft 4in and big with it, made his manipulative practice pretty impressive. Patients flocked to him and his healing rate was staggering. In his view the real element of the cure was the satisfying 'crack crack' as the back was deftly twisted, and he confided in me that to obtain the best results he always carried walnut shells in his pocket which he deftly crunched at the appropriate time to magnify the moment. Now that was healing.

Reference

1 Little P *et al.* (1997) Open randomised trial of prescribing strategies in managing sore throat. *British Medical Journal.* **314**: 722–7. (Follow up: *British Medical Journal.* **315**: 550–2.)

Chapter 18

Where from and where to?

My daughter is at the crossroads of her career and her life. She is about to enter the first pilot F2 year and is due to get married next May. She asked me recently what I thought of general practice as a job for life, and I found the answer difficult. Why? Because there are so many answers, and now I am at the opposite end of my career to hers my perspective is obviously very different. To her I am a wise-ish Dinosaur who happens to be her Dad, and I still see myself as a Young Turk. It is the mirror and the coronary arteries that tell a different story.

The truth, as you already know, is that general practice is entering one of its 'after the chrysalis' phases. We all know something new is hatching, we just don't know if it is a moth, a butterfly, or a Dodo destined for imminent extinction. I am reminded of the caterpillar looking up at the butterfly and announcing, 'You will never get me up in one of those things'.

Another truth that you already know is that some of the good things for patients and doctors are being lost. Continuity is the most important, probably, but loss of discretion over medical decisions comes pretty close. Protocols, electronic records, and multiple consultations with different professionals make it very very difficult to tailor the medicine to the patient, so we patients all have to buy off the peg; the days of bespoke doctoring are over. For many of us our suits don't fit too well and are not the style we would have chosen. In the great scheme of things this may not be too disastrous; at least we still have a suit, to continue the analogy.

When I started in general practice in 1972 a lot of practices and their practitioners were substandard; there were many reasons for this, including poor premises, poorly trained and poorly paid staff. Rotten record-keeping was the norm and the standard of the medicine purveyed was extremely varied. The patient experience, to quote a modern phrase, was extremely varied from Land's End to John O'Groats. Of course, it still is, but much less so. After a couple of government interventions things dramatically improved, and for a while a butterfly really did hatch, but it was relatively shortlived. Another hatching was precipitated by a new contract in the

1990s that also had fundholding tacked on to it. From my point of view this was a wonderful time. At last an ability to really act as the patient's advocate and bring real pressure to bear on secondary services to improve. But I was in the minority, the majority hated it and saw it as divisive, and this hatching turned into a Death's Head Moth. Fundholding is back again, of course, but in a more politically correct guise of BPC and without the useful bite of the earlier version. Vast polyclinics and big general practitioner-run A&Es look to be the mainstays of the future.

So what do I say to my daughter? Well, I could relate the family historical context and tell her about her grandfather and the hatchings he experienced.

'Four years after qualifying, at age 21 your grandfather took his MD by examination early in the Second World War. He passed but told me of the most difficult question he was asked: "What do you know about the aetiology of Crohn's disease?" He claimed he wrote, "I know very little about Crohn's disease at all". I mention this because if I were asked the same question today, more than 60 years later, my answer would be very similar. Medicine is advancing, but not as fast as society believes.

After the war, during which grandfather survived being torpedoed, bombed, etc., he joined up with Herbert Crisp as the junior partner in a general practice in South Shields. Herbert had been the family doctor forever; he had even delivered my father. In 1946, the year I was born, general practice was very different from now in so many ways. Perhaps the most important difference was the lack of clear split between hospital doctors and GPs. Your grandfather was a consulting physician to the Ingham Infirmary; he admitted patients there and looked after them in the hospital. He was also a surgeon if the need arose, and routinely took out tonsils at home. He used to do his own anaesthesia too. A terrifying thought to modern doctors. He was also a practising obstetrician, but his obstetrics was much more brutal and unforgiving than now. This was still an era when society accepted that childbearing was risky and that both mothers and children could, and not infrequently did, die. I still have a collection of his obstetric implements, tubes for puncturing heads to suck out brains to allow delivery and at least save the mother, a gadget to decapitate stuck babies, as well as the normal array of long, short and curved forceps. Herbert taught him to take a bucket with him when delivering a baby. The bucket was for drowning deformed babies. You may feel this description is unnecessarily frank, but medicine has always been brutal; there is an underlying rawness related to the struggles between life and death that our society does its best to screen us from.

In 1948, Aneurin Bevin imposed the National Health Service on an unwilling profession. Your grandfather hated the NHS, despised the British Medical Association for letting him down and felt betrayed for the rest of his career. He now had to make a decision he did not want to make, to stay in hospital or to make his life as a GP. Bevin had left no halfway house. Herbert was getting old and needed him, so in the end there was no choice. In order to make the new health service work, Bevin needed to get the powerful doctors on his side. He decided to pay generously those doctors remaining in hospital, the newly created 'consultants'. "I will stuff their mouths with gold", he is reputed to have said. He also encouraged contracts to allow private work to subsidise their earnings. The remaining GPs got none of this and became second-class citizens overnight. More than this, for most GPs their income dropped dramatically as traditional sources of income were subsumed by the hospitals. The day of the generalist was gone, specialism ruled. In 1952 Lord Moran, Churchill's physician, compounded the gloom for general practitioners by describing them as only those that had fallen off the hospital ladder. The only good doctors were in hospitals. The fact that this was unadulterated piffle has not stopped these beliefs being carried on to the present day, by hospital doctors and some of the public.

In the early 1950s a group of crusading GPs who cared about standards, academic rigour and, if the truth be stated, status formed a fledgling college that developed rapidly over the next decades to become the Royal College of General Practitioners (RCGP). One of the founders, William Pickles, a GP from Wensleydale, had done some wonderful rigorous and beautifully simple research into the spread of infectious disease in Yorkshire villages. His biography remains in print and at some stage you should read it. It is a great testament to the generalist. Anecdotally, I shared a study with his grandson when I was a pupil at Giggleswick School in Yorkshire. Your grandfather did not think much of the new college, being convinced it was a clique-driven, status-seeking exercise, peopled by pompous windbags bent on self-aggrandisement. He was wrong, I think, but the College too is at a crossroads, a new exam will soon replace the old, standards will change and if the College won't make a stand for quality and standards then its very purpose becomes unclear. But I digress.

The gloom years of general practice lasted from the late 1940s until the mid-1960s, then an imaginative Charter set about improving premises and working conditions. The RCGP set up vocational training and instituted an examination. From the early 1970s to the mid-1980s the best medical school graduates went into general practice, metaphorically waving the famous Agincourt salute to Lord Moran. Grandfather died, still working singlehandedly, in 1975 of myasthenia gravis. Your grandmother was still his receptionist and his premises were awful, but his patients loved him and too many people came for them all to get into his funeral.

I was a course organiser in the late 1970s and there were 10–20 applicants for every place on my scheme at that time. By the year 2000 there was fewer than one. It is picking up again, however, probably because of the major change in the service commitment. For many new entrants it is a 9–5 job that is extremely well paid and with no night duty; this is an attractive if very different animal from the one I remember.

So what should you do, O daughter of mine? Raising a family is certainly easier in practice than in hospital, and what do you want from your career? Is it a job or a vocation? I think I should tell you about the real joys of general practice, but I will save that for next time.'

Chapter 19

Waving not drowning

Now where was I? Ah yes; the real joys of general practice. Bear with me and I will get there eventually. Nearly three years ago I was driving through my patch and I waved at a patient of many years' standing who I had not seen for some time, forgetting one of the cardinal GP rules; *never* wave at a patient as they will invariably appear in the surgery within the next 24 hours. He did, it was complicated and emotionally involving in a draining sort of way, and I really wished I hadn't waved. At the time I was already a bit poorly, and very soon afterwards I became ill. Our patients learn pretty quickly that major illness alters their perspective on life, its value, its length and its meaning; it was a lesson I still had to learn. Two years ago I wrote about my own experience of major illness in myself and my wife. Sadly she died, but I survived: now enough time has passed to gain some perspective for myself. This series of cardiac events, pacemaker wire infection leading to endocarditis and the discovery of rotten arteries necessitating a quadruple graft suddenly and unexpectedly tipped me out of my familiar job of 30 years, and after some time in hospital I sort of surfaced, retired, widowed and disorientated. I could have added depressed too, but on reflection I wasn't. I was unhappy and lonely, and both emotions were both necessary and justified, and both were normal, but there was no-one to wave at any more. My waved-at patient did send me a get well card.

So what good things did I miss about being a GP? Well, first and foremost the biggest miss was the company, my medical partners, the health centre staff and my patients, not in any particular order. Company in this context means someone to talk to, to listen to, to share, to help and to be helped by. I became aware of what a tremendously supportive environment I had sort of taken for granted. Is it as good in hospital? I doubt it.

I missed my registrar, both in general and in particular. This is a special relationship, dear old Eric Berne's transactional analysis doesn't quite cope with it. It is not quite adult/adult, but it's not parent/child, though sometimes it is probably closest to enquiring child/child relationships. It had always been clear to me that I had probably got more out of my one-to-one teacher/pupil relationships than I put in; there was always the underlying feeling of guilt at enjoying this more than one was supposed to, like sipping at a delicious and forbidden elixir of youth garnished, like a Pimms, with fresh raw experience and new untried knowledge, while pretending to one's partners that it was only warm beer in a plastic cup. Then I missed having something regular to do, and a tiny bit of security evaporated, and the little worm began the journey into the apple of self-worth.

I did and do still have an appointment, as convenor of the RCGP Panel of Examiners. This is not a job in the normal sense, there being no salary, no regular hours, an unclear and ever-changing job description, and almost no yardsticks with which to measure success or failure. Some candidates will not empathise with this remark. Needless to say, in a time of personal crisis so it is with GP assessment, the old is going, the new is coming and there is no stopping it. Perhaps this is a case of the wrong man, in the wrong place at the wrong time, because I do regret the passing of the old and the over-hasty adoption of the new, but then, as Mandy Rice Davies so famously said when the cabinet minister denied, on oath, having sex with her, 'Well, he would wouldn't he!'.

The reason I bring this up, as it were, in the context of good things I miss is to highlight the importance of good effective communication being in the repertoire of the modern doctor. Conversations with patients are a GP's lifeblood; transfused back to the patients, it can be theirs too. I was one of a group that took the challenge on, over 15 years ago now, to develop an examination of doctors' consulting ability; we used videotape, as it was the most useful methodology of the time. The first and overriding aim of this assessment was to put consulting on the academic map, to make it important enough for doctors to study it and practise it. In other words, the exam was primarily intended to drive learning. Well, as you know we didn't get it all right, the methodology was clunky, the criteria seemed clumsy to some, and some behaviours were selectively, if accidentally, overused. 'Are you worried that you are the man who put options into general practice?' asked a weary colleague after watching yet another spurious offering of non-realistic alternatives to a bemused patient.

Now, what I really miss is the teaching of how to consult more effectively with my own registrars, and I still think the video (soon to be DVD) examination is a good but more importantly a necessary test. I also firmly believe that the current MRCGP examination is a good package, if lacking a good simulated case-controlled clinical element, but in an educational somersault of breathtaking suddenness, soon that is all the assessment will be, a newly developed simulation plus the MCQ.

The real reason I am going on about communication, discourse, chat, whatever, is that I have rediscovered what fun it is and have been reminded how privileged we doctors are. You see, my life got better: I remarried, moved to deepest Dorset and unpacked the stethoscope on a very part-time basis, started seeing patients again and, this is not flannel, what a joy it was.

There are some guilty secrets amongst my recent discoveries, however. One is that continuity is not an unmixed blessing, for doctor or patient. After 30 years attitudes have fixed, ears have closed and patterns have become preordained; being able to recite the probable patients and their complaints for one's evening surgery before even looking is an amusing game to entertain bored receptionists, but perhaps symptomatic of a developing malaise. I confess to never knowing patients as well as they thought I did, and sometimes after 30 years of regular contact my knowledge of the real life of that human being in front of me was pathetic.

This was starkly demonstrated some years ago. The police interviewed me about a tragic murder of a respectable lady patient. What could I tell them? Well, very little, as it transpired, despite seeing her regularly for several years. What was her job, they asked? Shop assistant, I say. Yes, yes, but what did I know about her real job? Her real job? I ask with furrowed brow and quizzical expression. Yes doc, of course you knew she was on the game, didn't you? Well, no I didn't, though it transpired nearly everyone else in the town did. This has remained a salutary lesson to me. People tell you what they want you to hear. Sometimes with skill and curiosity you get a bit deeper, but after a while it becomes difficult to ask the deeper questions and the relationship skates along fairly superficially unless there is a major disturbance. Record-keeping in this litigious age has become precise, detailed and much better than it was, but there is little or no time for social recording, and it could be that knowing about one's patients will become harder, not easier.

It was with this increasingly sceptical view that I nervously took up the stethoscope again. After 30 years of developing expertise, writing books, pontificating, running examinations, that night I lay awake listening to the clock strike the quarters before my first surgery for nearly three years, wondering if I could still consult adequately; and then I started seeing patients again, new patients, new stories, new surgery, it was wonderful. No baggage, no preconceptions, clean slate, just like my registrars, it was and is invigorating. This is heresy, but I now believe we should all change practice every five to ten years for the benefit of ourselves and our patients.

I quite liked the maligned QOF, the recording discipline helped jog the clinical brain cells and it was not as intrusive as the detractors would have you believe. The time pressures were better than where I had been working, I could and did say 'tell me more' and mean it. The patients did, and I was fascinated.

Visiting an old people's home to see a lady with chronic constipation and dementia would have been a downer in my last life. Now the sun was shining, here was the sea, the cliffs of the Isle of Wight clearly visible and the old lady told me a Hardyesque tale of a childhood in rural Dorset. She tells it to everyone, but the first time it is still fresh and interesting. I drive back, I wave at a new dimly recognised acquaintance, I wave at another and another, soon I could give the Queen lessons. This time I hope they *will* come to see me.

Chapter 20

Measureless to man?

There are not many things that human beings agree about. This is so self-evident it hardly needs stating. In fact, offhand, I can't think of anything that every human being would agree about. The more complex the thought or task, the more the opinions and disagreements; as an illustration we could start with God and whether he or she exists, etc., but where would that get us? Except perhaps to a sudden extermination by a fellow human who feels and thinks differently. It would, of course, help if there were universal truths and laws. This is already a matter for disagreement, as some people think there are; you will have gathered that I am not in that particular camp. Let me go back to medicine. There are certainly no universal truths there, except possibly that whatever today's most popular treatments are, they will be tomorrow's amusing little anecdotes contained in a small box in the bowels of the *British Medical Journal*. If there is a God, it would have been very helpful for the deity to produce a manual on all of Earth's creatures, particularly Mrs It's-my-funny-turns-again from No. 30. I could then look up the appropriate entry on 'funny turns', read the FAQs and look at the suggested solutions, just like I can for my car, washing machine, etc. On reflection, having a manual without the skill to really use it is not such a step forward, but it would be of some help in cutting the level of disagreement between Mrs Imfta and me. This lack of a personal manual bedevils medicine, generalisations must rule, epidemiology guides the thought processes, and trial results on different people leading different lives have to guide how I try to help Mrs Imfta. If I write up Mrs Imfta's case for an article and ask for suggestions and opinions, there will be a good response, but these suggestions and opinions will all be different. This is from a learned profession all apparently trained, assessed and examined in the discipline. Here is a truth: training does not produce agreement.

Perversely, with a lot of our examinations the reverse seems to apply; there is almost universal agreement, but it is not very helpful agreement. As I write, it is A-level time again. A leading private school has found that 95% of its entrants have As or A+s, the tabloids are bleating 'what sort of exam is this?' and the universities really have no idea who to choose. The pupils in the Sixth Form, however, have a much better idea who is any good and who isn't, and could give you a much better rank ordering than the exam results. In the bad old days of the 11-plus, just one mark could make the difference between a successful life or a blighted one, and this was what ultimately probably did for that examination. The pass/fail border is always uncomfortable territory in exams that matter, and of course, it is here that the paths are most blurred, and it is easy to stray into the wrong territory. There are no easy answers to this dilemma; the A-level solution of passing nearly everybody is not helpful, but the alternative of failing the wrong people is a worry too. The restructuring of the GP assessment process may produce a system that could fall into the A-level trap, but there is no doubt that the current MRCGP examination, which is quite hard, is sometimes perceived as harsh by aggrieved candidates who fell the wrong side of the cutting edge. Many such candidates write in to me expressing disgruntlement and often citing opinions from respected colleagues who disagree with the examination verdict. On nearly all such occasions, investigations of such queries reveal the candidate to be very near the necessarily arbitrary pass/fail divide, but of course on the wrong side of it. Candidates usually seek advice on how this state of affairs can be rectified. My predecessor as convenor of the MRCGP, Roger Neighbour, suggested the blindingly obvious strategy of 'try doing better next time!', as this remark in fact points out that the best way to be certain of passing a difficult examination is to be a good candidate and so avoid the murky waters of the pass/fail divide.

Some exams are reputedly more reliable than others, with the computer-marked MCQ type being singled out for particular reverence. There is a lot of evidence that the results of such tests are in fact very reproducible, but always the sneaking worry that it is quite possible to be reliably wrong. A good friend tells of the time he visited a distinguished medical royal college and heard a plethora of angry voices raised as he passed a large, book-lined room. Who were these angry men, so plainly and vociferously disagreeing? He was told they were the senior examiners discussing the correct answers for the next MCQ.

Assessors are needed at every stage of an assessment process, and who should take on this task? In general practice there is now an industry churning out assessors of all sorts, and some have this burden thrust upon them, trainers being the obvious example. The core of the current and future summative assessment will be the trainers' report, and there is plenty of evidence, actual and anecdotal, that many trainers are not good at actually assessing the relative strengths and weaknesses of their registrars. Some of the angriest letters of the 'How dare you fail my registrar, who is the best we have ever seen, etc.' type turn out to be about candidates who have in fact done very badly indeed. Somebody is wrong, and an examination that samples widely and with a measurable degree of reliability is in this situation more likely to be nearer the truth. But assessing is difficult; doctors who put themselves forward to be examiners for the MRCGP have to go through a stringent selection process, looking for aptitude, knowledge, trainability, group skills and, most importantly, the ability to rank order. It is this latter skill that is most crucial, as experience has shown that those who do not have the innate ability to rank order, or in basic terms the ability to distinguish pillar-boxes from elephants, good consulters from bad, bullshitters from truthsayers, cannot be trained to develop this skill. Most, but not all, children have this innate ability, which is why they are often better judges of their colleagues than the examinations are. Those who do not have this ability should not be selected as assessors.

The ability of oral examiners for the MRCGP serves as an example of some of the differing skills needed by assessors; a good oral examiner needs to develop the ability to ask easy-to-understand but searching questions that test the candidate in an immediate and intimate interview style. In other words, the assessor must have the skill to efficiently generate the material to be judged. The next, and equally important, skill is actually making the judgement. Good assessors do both, but there are many variations on a theme. There are waffly examiners, who seem to make good judgements on thin material; and there are the extremely waspish, thorough and inquisitive types, who then make rather bland middle-of-the-road judgements; and there is the opposite, the iron fist in the velvet glove. Assessors have classically been divided into hawks and doves, and in the MRCGP examination these tendencies are noted and attempts are made to cancel out the effects of such intrinsic human behaviour, by detailed standard setting meetings for the written examination, and adjustment of groups for the oral and video modules.

To go back to what I intended the point of this article to be, wide-ranging agreement is not a common human characteristic, but good postgraduate medical assessment requires it, so not everyone will be able to do it. Criteria can help, but agreeing them in the first place and then recognising what was agreed is not easy. Just think about 'Dr picks up cues'; almost total agreement that this seemed a necessary criterion to demonstrate consulting competence, but very little agreement about what this apparently simple and unequivocal statement actually meant. Some truths must now be apparent; all future assessors of doctors must be selected for aptitude, and especially an ability to rank order candidates in the particular area of their assessment. They must be trained and their own performance assessed, and there must be a system of review and revalidation. The tests themselves must be scrutinised, and here there may be educational compromises. Some tests may be less reliable, but more educationally constructive, so a policy of not putting all one's eggs in one basket would seem a wise maxim. Any test of a future doctor's ability should be wide ranging, sampling in many areas, and be a mix of assessment methodologies. They won't all agree, but a summation will be a fairer measure than an individual result. It may not be Coleridge's stately pleasure dome, but it may be that man can get a reasonable measure before disappearing into a sunless sea.

Chapter 21

Good points first

I have to confess a secret addiction to reality TV programmes. You know the sort, groups of strange young men pretending to be legionnaires or very unpleasant yobettes trying to be ladies, etc. Recently I watched a series called *The Unteachables* about the most unruly and difficult young teenagers the TV company could lay their hands on being collected together and sent to an outward-bound school with the best teachers they could find. The results were mixed and on the whole very heartening, but what really hit home was a picture of the most difficult of the pupils not to have been actually thrown out, convulsed in uncontrollable sobbing at the end of the penultimate programme. Why was this? Had he been beaten? Had he been expelled at the last? No, he had just read his detailed report. So it was bad then? No, it was good. So why the sobbing? asked the presenter. He managed to stutter out that this was the first time anyone had ever said anything good about him. 'I am happy and I am upset', he actually said. The next week they gave him a young class to teach by himself. At the end of the excellent lesson he singled out the three weakest pupils and praised them in front of their form mates; it was inspirational, humbling and it took me 20 minutes to get the lump out of my throat.

Now, to get to be a doctor, many people must have said pretty good things about you, but at medical school, and certainly in the earlier years of hospital students, young medics tend to get cut back to size. The self-doubt creeps back in, we get used to a point-scoring, adversarial, oneupmanship style of teaching. You have to know one more syndrome than your colleague, think of the blood test no one else has thought of, and to take pretty fierce criticism on the chin. Some years ago, a young nervous student was having the mysteries of a diabetic retinitis demonstrated by an aggressive and impatient chief. The student had not fully grasped the skills of ophthalmoscopy, but was desperately trying to maintain some personal credibility with his irascible tutor. 'Well, what do you see?' To all observing, including the chief, the ophthalmoscope light was now brightly illuminating a patch of pillow to the left of the patient's head and it was obvious that the young man was not seeing anything of the retina. Gamely, but unwisely, he continued, giving a fictitious description of what he was not yet skilled enough to see. The chief bellowed at him, 'You silly little worm, if you had an IQ of one less you would be a plant . . .'. This form of constructive feedback is not likely to make us keen to reveal our innermost secrets to a group of doctors; like our unteachable friend, we can begin to lose faith in ourselves and begin to think we really are hopeless, and what is worse is that we can begin to act like it.

You can sense that I am edging nearer to Pendleton's rules; just a reminder of the simplest version.

- **Rule 1. Good points first.**
- **Rule 2. No criticism without recommendation.**

Let me tell you my version of how they came into being. In 1979 I took extended study leave to work with a charismatic evangelical young man who had arrived in Oxford with a mission to influence patient–doctor communication. I had been a course organiser in Oxford for a year and my own inexperience and ignorance of the human condition, let alone teaching ability, were being systematically exposed. I was also still coming to terms with my own mortality, mixed with surprise at how uninvolved in my fears my doctors were; this was my second year with a cardiac pacemaker and I was just the wrong side of 30. David Pendleton was preaching that doctors should understand their patient's fears and that communication with patients should be taught as a priority, second only to a good medical education. I wanted this personally and at last saw a teaching focus that I could really engage with. So, like many motives, mine were fundamentally self-centred, and as a result all the more powerful.

The Department of Experimental Psychology, the ugliest building in Oxford, was filled with fascinating people at that time. Michael Argyll, the doyen of social skills, who would never look you in the eye, the Peters Marsh and Collett, still to be regularly found on our TV screens, Adrian Furnham, the charismatic and very media friendly soon to be a professor at UCL, and many others. In the next door Department of Zoology the great man-watcher and postural echoer, Desmond Morris, had his lair. The place was buzzing and it was very easy to feel both inferior and out of one's depth, which I did. One morning, early in my stay, a very glamorous, hard-edged Brisbanian called Monica entered our dark, bare breeze-blocked cell without so much as a knock. I was conspicuously alone.

'You seen Pendleton?' 'Er no.' 'Know where he is?' 'Er no.' 'Jees, I wouldn't pee in your ear if your brains were on fire.'

So this was academia. 'Monica doesn't take prisoners,' was David's initial contribution. 'I wouldn't like her to criticise my consultations,' said I, desultorily shuffling a pile of black-and-white reel-to-reel videotapes of just that. 'Well, it would be a bracing experience,' said DP, 'but probably not a constructive one.' So Monica was the seed; how could we discuss something as sensitive, personal and vulnerable as consulting without it turning into a destructive disaster? We kept coming back to this crux. Peter Havelock and Theo Schofield were course organisers too and all three of us were trying to teach consulting on our respective Thames Valley vocational training courses. In the car one day Bing Crosby sang about accentuating the positive and eliminating the negative and a few conversations and a seminar later we got the rules, the principle being to teach from observed strengths, so building confidence and fostering the creation of a milieu conducive to learning sensitive skills. In young and inexperienced hands like mine this produced a whole new style of teaching, described by DP after watching one of my VTS seminars as 'hitting the learner with the carrot'.

At the same time the department was seething with attribution theory, why people in various circumstances did what they did. We looked at patients, opened the suitcase labelled 'Health Beliefs', and out popped 'Ideas, Concerns and Expectations' (ICE). A mnemonic that launched a thousand courses was born. This was 26 years ago as I write; my daughter was born at precisely this time, which locks the date in my mind. The four of us are still proud of these contributions, ICE and the rules, and of the books these ideas spawned, and perhaps more importantly of the behaviours they changed and the patients who benefited. Of course, ICE has become trite and oft trotted out without thinking, let alone being put into practice, and the rules have been modified and changed by many. This has also spawned new terms such as 'The Blodgit', being the standard unit of insincere praise, and 'The Shit Sandwich', indicating that if you are not careful everything before the 'but what could you have done better?' is bullshit. Only integrity, honesty and practice can get rid of this, otherwise the exercise can and does degenerate into a sham.

Those early days of good points first were, however, revelatory, after the traditional response to the question of 'what did you do well?', which was a slow flapping motion of the hands with a silent open and closing of the mouth, well described as the Goldfish response. The groups of young doctors were soon spectacularly good at recognising effective skills in their colleagues without, in the vast majority of cases, being insincere or glutinous. Of course, doctors do like being criticised a bit, and they like the sensation of learning spiced with a bit of mustard sometimes, but the environment has to be safe to allow this to happen and we soon discovered that if we did let the rules relax too much, learners were hurt and the learning suffered. This is still true. We have run some very successful courses totally based on only positive feedback and constructive sugges-tions reinforced by role-play; Bing would have been pleased at the elimination of the negative.

So have we influenced GPs' behaviour for the good over this quarter of a century? You will have to be the judge of that; we know some schemes have wriggled clear of the rules and some have modified and replaced them with thoughtful descriptive scenarios, but the underlying idea remains the same – emphasise the positive. Not all medical education appears to have moved on, some is still very adversarial and sometimes belittling, but this appears to be a weakening trend; in fact, emphasising the positive is not a bad recipe for struggling through this life. Now with the whole new educational system for doctors in the process of rapid, almost bewildering, change, we know this is a time when lots of babies can be swept out into the sewage amongst the copious old bathwater being discarded, which means that this, more than ever, is a time to emphasise the positive. Oh Peter, tell me what you think about the new reforms, with particular emphasis on the work-based assessments . . . Good points first!

Chapter 22

The Pharaoh

By the 1960s the British Raj was a rapidly fading communal memory of thick ruby port voices on late-night radio programmes discussing tiger shoots. The subcontinent was divided into the two Pakistans, East and West, Muslim in creed, with India in the middle, now populated mainly by Hindus and Sikhs. Independence had been granted as recently as 1947, but the only legacies remaining to the average Englishman were dark curry houses with furry wallpaper and golden elephants on the walls, and the National Health Service. At this juncture in history, all general hospitals in ordinary unglamorous towns were staffed almost exclusively by doctors from the subcontinent. The plum consultant jobs were still mostly in the hands of UK graduates, but the senior registrar, registrar, senior house officer and houseman posts were 95% Asian. The British graduates clustered into the teaching hospitals, the centres of excellence, bastions of privilege and prejudice, where dark faces were rarely seen and then only at monthly district meetings.

The South Shields General Hospital was an old workhouse. It was not in any way glamorous and it had only one white houseman – me. My father was a general practitioner in the town, and it was his longstanding friendship with a local surgeon that had led me back to the old hospital to be apprenticed to him for six months. It was the time of the war between India and Pakistan over disputed areas of Kashmir, and the mix of doctors then working in the hospital was approximately two-thirds Pakistani and one-third Indian. Relationships were fraught and tension was high. This was not helped by the communal living arrangements of the doctors. We were all obliged to live in a self-contained stockade-like edifice situated a hundred yards from the main hospital and known to all as 'The Ranch.'

As the tension built up, the rival groups tried to cope by enlisting humour, but religious and patriotic rivalry is no laughing matter, and the two groups quickly polarised absolutely into separate dissenting factions with an attitude of mutual loathing. The demarcation of living-room space and use of dinner tables became rigid, with unspoken but unbreakable rules that were clearly understood by all. The various medical and surgical teams began to suffer, especially those with a religious mix, intermediaries such as myself passed messages and many jobs went undone. To make matters worse, each faction followed the daily news of the war in the newspapers and on the BBC news bulletins with a fanatical intensity, celebrating successes without restraint, each time increasing the gap between them and raising the level and intensity of the recriminations.

During this period there were only three non-combatants living in the Ranch – myself (a wet-behind-the-ears agnostic Geordie), Freddie (a Patan from Afghanistan whose father was a chief, while he was heir apparent) and Khurshid Qasimayya (a young Egyptian doctor with a physique like a Nubian wrestler and a similar command of the English language). In the early stages of the conflict it was Freddie who helped most. He had no truck with either India or Pakistan. His revered forebears had a long and proud record of fighting all comers, from Alexander the Great to the British (and of course more recently the Russians, the Americans and the British again), and it was his solemn boast that although his fierce tribesmen had occasionally lost a skirmish, they had never truly lost a war.

Freddie was a wiry dark aquiline man with thick black grizzled hair, and quick searching eyes that demonstrated to those who wished to see them glimpses of his cat-like intelligence and warrior's rumbustious sense of humour, unusual on the subcontinent. In keeping with his persona he was possessed of an acute awareness of the feelings of others, detecting subtle nuances where others would just see hatred. If Freddie followed a God he never told the rest of us, but he did attempt to stop the others being consumed by their own Gods. He seemed to decide that if he could not stop the real war, he could at least help to make the war that was being waged in this little part of Tyneside look as ridiculous to the combatants as it did to the onlookers. He set about regaling each side systematically with blood-chilling tales of his people's sufferings, their massacres, their triumphs and their many pyrrhic victories. He adjusted the tales only a little depending on his audience. To the Indians he described the deeds of his warriors against the Sikhs and the Hindus, and to the Pakistanis he recounted their deeds against the Muslims of the plain. Always of course the Patans were superior in every department, one musket- and knife-wielding terror from the mountains bettering at least ten Indians or Pakistanis in every bloody encounter, always out-generalling and out-lasting their puny opponents.

Initially irritation was the dominant emotion in the opposing camps when Freddie tried his simple strategy, but gradually his humour, his persistence and his underlying sense of the ridiculous, backed by centuries of futile suffering, began to tell on the entrenched belligerence of the two sides. The atmosphere became less charged, even an occasional smile could be seen, and jokes in football metaphors began to appear along the lines of 'India 2, Pakistan 1, but it's gone to extra time.' The mess was still not a pleasant place in which to live, but Freddie had made it bearable.

Khurshid, the Egyptian, was an altogether different kettle of fish. He was one of those human beings who is forever doomed to be in the wrong place at the wrong time, doing the wrong thing for the wrong reasons. In a brief acquaintance this can be an almost endearing trait, but living with such a ninny, especially one with no command of the language of the land, could become somewhat trying. He was not helped by his choice of South Tyneside as his little part of England in which to stay and gain experience – an area with distinct customs and an impenetrable dialect that could only be understood by true natives, born-and-bred Geordies. The Geordies are by and large a good-natured, wry-humoured group who could not cope easily with a name like Khurshid Qasimayya, so within no time after his arrival at the hospital he was christened 'The Pharaoh' (Fair-O in the dialect).

Within a few days of his starting to work as a front-of-house casualty officer, Khurshid was confronted by a distraught young father who pulled him into a cubicle with the following desperate message: 'Docta, Docta, kum quick like. Wor bairn's fair felled an he's gorra load of blebs under his oxters an' he's burnin' up. Wor hen's beside hersel' with frit.'

One week's study of colloquial English at the South Tyne Polytechnic was insufficient for Khurshid to have even the faintest clue what the father was talking about. A large world-weary casualty sister of the type they sadly don't seem to make any more translated slowly for him.

'What Mr Jones is trying to tell you, Doctor, is that he is worried about his little boy, who has a rash of spots under his armpits and who seems to have a high temperature. His wife is very worried, too. I think he has a mild dose of the chickenpox.' Khurshid only lasted six months, as you will find out, but his English never did improve, forever held back by the vernacular. He must have returned to his ancient homeland with confused tales of this strange tribe of people living on the banks of a famous river, whose customs and language were indecipherable to civilised nations. Perhaps he had unwittingly discovered how the Emperor Hadrian probably felt.

The Geordie people had a deeply schizophrenic view of the foreign doctors who were entrusted to look after them. They saw themselves as a separate tribe that just happened to live in North-East England, so to some extent the Indians, Pakistanis and even the Pharaoh were acknowledged as members of just another tribe, like Scotsmen or Scousers or even Brummies. It was the older people whose deeply entrenched small-town racism proved a greater barrier to communication with the foreign doctors than any language barrier. My great aunt Vera was one of these. At the time of this story she was 80 years old, a small wizened spinster who had been a ladies' hatter in the town for 50 years, a business she had run with her eccentric sister Nellie. Neither of them had married, as both had lost their future husbands on the Somme and had accepted that marriage was not for them. Rarely did any man venture into their little powdered shop, and those who did were soon shooed away. Vera, the last and tiniest of a family of 15, was known colloquially as 'the poke shakings', and had her left kidney removed on the kitchen table in extremely primitive and unhygienic circumstances at the age of five. The doctor had solemnly given her but a few weeks to live. However, Vera did not have another day's illness until her eightieth year, demonstrating clearly the medical profession's fallibility when predicting the future.

Pain in the lower part of her belly and a fear of dying had brought great aunt Vera into South Shields General Hospital. She had lasted for a week at home, but the onset of vomiting and a complete blockage of the bowel finally ended her resistance, and now she lay clutching the sheet to her chin and peering fiercely at the group of doctors at the foot of her bed. The tale was related to me later by Freddie the Patan, the senior surgical registrar. The Pharaoh was cowering at the back of the group as far away from the old woman as he could get while still maintaining contact with the ward round.

'Stay away, the lot of you' squawked an obviously cornered Vera. 'It's not yer faces I object to, it's yer black hands, and *him*.' A white stick-like arm shot out from under the sheet and pointed unequivocally at the cowering Pharaoh, 'He's a menace, a loony. He's not a doctor, he's a monkey, all he talks is gibberish and he tried to stick a needle into my belly. Well, I'm not having it and that's final.' She pulled the sheet even tighter to her chin and glowered at the assembled group, daring them to make a move. Freddie took a pace forward, and Vera shrank away up on her pillow.

'Gerroff.' It was a stand-off.

Freddie turned to the ward sister for an explanation of the old woman's aggression towards Dr Qasimayya, not wishing to risk a long incoherent conversation with the man himself. Sister cast her eyes heavenwards.

'I am afraid neither Miss Scarfe nor Dr Qasimayya understood much of what the other said. Miss Scarfe objected to him trying to examine her, and screamed out loud when he put his hand on her tummy. I believe this somewhat unnerved Dr Qasimayya, for when he tried to take some blood from Miss Scarfe's arm he tripped, yelled, and stabbed the syringe into her just below the umbilicus. Miss Scarfe became hysterical, called him a screaming dervish, and demonstrated a command of explicit vocabulary surprising in an elderly spinster. Fortunately I don't believe Dr Qasimayya understood any of it, but I suspect he got the drift. Unfortunately, Miss Scarfe has not let anyone near her since, including my nurses, so something will have to be done.'

The assembled group looked at one another, while Vera's steel blue eyes moved from left to right and back again, strafing the lot of them. Even Freddie flinched. The Pharaoh pointed both his arms to the ceiling and then thrust them apart in a gesture of despair, or perhaps it was prayer, while mumbling something incomprehensible to the assembled gathering.

'See, see, he's gibbering, what did I tell you? Off his trolley he is. I came in to be cured and all I get is attacked by a mad gippo and stared at by a bunch of darkies.' Vera leaned back on her pillow, and the sickness and the pain began to cloud her previously clear eyes. Freddie the compassionate humorist saw his chance, adopted his Peter Sellars imitation of Indian dialect, and spoke with exaggerated formality to this prickly but frightened Geordie great aunt.

'My good white woman, I am the son of a chief, mine is a fierce warlike tribe, we are cannibals, too.' He paused for effect, and Vera's pupils dilated a little. 'We enjoy eating white men, cooking them slowly in hot stones, but the greatest delicacy is the white woman.' He leaned forward quickly and Vera shut her eyes. 'So tender, so delicate, so aromatic. It is the meat from the palm of the hand that is the sweetest. Ah, the memories of those good dinners come flooding back to me.' Freddie was holding the old lady's hand now and smiled at her. There was a long silence. Vera slowly opened her eyes and stared at the Afghan Prince, and then she smiled.

'Eeeh, you're havin' me on.' She looked hard at Freddie to be sure, and he just carried on smiling. 'Perhaps yer alreet after all, me nephew said you were a good 'un, if it's you to do it gan on, dee what you have to dee and let's be done with it.' She let go of the sheet and was a model patient from then on. The operation to remove a large colonic polyp was a success, and she cheated the great reaper again, but she would not let the Pharaoh near her.

Vera did have to stay in the hospital for several weeks, and her already run down bungalow assumed an air of dereliction and neglect. The evening of her discharge, some local youths decided that it looked a good bet for a spot of pillage and vandalism. It was round about eleven at night when they broke in, and the mustiness and the cold confirmed their belief that the place was empty, so they made no attempt to be quiet. Vera was awakened from her light post-hospital slumber by the sound of these three lads rummaging about in the Ottoman trunk at the end of her bed. Ever a courageous old bird, she sat bolt upright in the moonlit gloom. With no wig on, so no hair, no teeth and in a shroud-like old lace nightie, she yelled at her burglars in a high-pitched crackly voice 'So what do ye lot think you're doin'? Gerrout or I'll set the dogs on ye all.' The fact that she had never owned more than a Pekinese in her whole life was of little interest to the terrified marauders. This ghastly spectre so unnerved them that they fled as if all the hounds of hell were snapping at their heels. I doubt whether they ever continued with a life of crime, although possibly one of them, haunted by such a vision in his formative years, became a video producer for Michael Jackson.

Back at the Ranch an uneasy truce prevailed. The open hostility had gone, but the tension was palpable, and mealtimes were especially difficult. The two staff were determined to improve this state of affairs. The main entrance to the doctors' quarters was via a cluttered old Victorian-style kitchen, full of hanging pots, a boiled cabbage smell, large knives with ground-down blades, and unidentifiable bubbling concoctions on various gas rings. The staff consisted of Madge the cook and Ena who dealt with everything else. Madge was short and round, with a figure like a prehistoric fertility goddess and an outrageous opinion on any topic. She seemed to live at the Ranch. Although she had a family of six teenagers, she never seemed to go home. Neither did Ena, who was a tall, bottle blonde and always wore bright red lipstick and lots of mascara. Like Madge she was probably about 45 years old, but it was not easy to tell. She was childless but apparently happily married to a husband no one ever saw. The two of them never stopped talking, arguing and often shouting. It was like the Duchess and the Cook in *Alice in Wonderland*, but with the roles reversed.

Madge, like most people on South Tyneside, was a rabid socialist by declaration, but with such right-wing views as to make the then topical Enoch Powell look moderate. She loved goading the foreign doctors with downright racist remarks, delivered in a rumbustious 'like it or lump it' style that made any limp liberal unused to her behaviour wince with pain and embarrassment, although Madge saw herself as a gentle tease with a heart of gold. Ena was the appeaser, who would try to excuse Madge's more outrageous utterances and tone down her milder jibes with soothing excuses to the audience, which of course only provoked Madge to go one better. The whole dialogue usually took place among the steam and strange cooking smells, where figures could appear and disappear in quite an eerie fashion, and the grin of the Cheshire cat would not have seemed incongruous.

For their part, the insulted doctors began to try to exchange banter in kind, as a defence mechanism, so conversations usually took the form of mutually escalating insults that were frequently interrupted by Ena's high-pitched 'Eeeh, you mustna say that, that's aawful.' Madge, for all her vitriol, was essentially good humoured, and most exchanges ended in laughter plus a final stinging Parthian shot from the steamy mist.

The mixed religions of the subcontinent were ignored altogether by Madge in her menu construction. She cooked an unending sequence of dumplings, steak and kidney pie and pudding, stewed cabbage and corned beef fritters with mashed potato, followed by treacle tart or semolina pudding. She never seemed to notice or care that this fare was less than rapturously received. It was good enough for her own menfolk so it was good enough for the foreigners. Freddie realised that his tale-telling stratagem was losing its effectiveness, and decided that perhaps an attack on the menu would be a powerful unifying force. By making remarks here and there over a period of a week or so he managed to foment a reasonably good-natured revolution, and as the opposing camps drew together in condemnation of the uninspiring diet that was being foisted upon them, gradually the temperature of the exchanges rose.

'Hey, Madge, what about a decent curry?'

'Why, that's nasty hot stuff, ruins good meat, only daft foreigners would eat that muck.'

'Eeeh, you mustna say that.'

'Well, I say warra I mean, youse lot are in England now and you should eat wor fud, when in Rome they say.'

'Yes, Madge, but we are not in Rome. A pizza or a spaghetti bolognese would be good, but a curry would be best. We would even cook it ourselves.'

'Over my dead body, none of youse lot is setting a paw in my kitchen.' Madge looked defiantly at the seated doctors with plates of only slightly nibbled corn beef fritters, and sensed a tide that she had not experienced before, a feeling of genuine rebellion.

Ena broke the deadlock: 'Aw, gan on Madge, you show em, make em a Madge special curry.'

'Yes, go on Madge, make us a special curry, cheer us all up.'

Madge made her mind up, 'OK hinnies, I'll show you buggers what a curry should really be like. I'll bet I can make a canny curry, better than any of youse lot. Ye better put the bog roll in fridge now because you'll need it.'

Having picked up the gauntlet she was determined to put on a good show, and even more determined to show her doctors that she really was a cosmopolitan cook, and that the regular fritters were due to economics and not to lack of inspiration or skill (or to the fact that half the doctors' budget was probably siphoned off to feed her own family). She rummaged through her cupboards, and raided the main hospital stores for any spices, raisins, lentils and rice that could be found. One morning the Pharaoh met her coming to work with a large brown paper parcel and a smile of defiant satisfaction on her face. She beamed at him and patted her parcel: 'Abdulla from Chi's best hot curry powder, all the chillies in the East in this stuff, blow the arse off that Sphinx of yours, guaranteed five-star bum burner.' The Pharaoh smiled at her uncomprehendingly and offered 'You soon to make good curry, I look it forward, you best cook Madge.'

As you may already have gathered, Madge suffered from the widespread Northern delusion that for a curry to be any good it had to lift off the top of the head while simultaneously shrivelling the tonsils. Subtle nuances of flavour were not for her – this was heroic cookery.

At last the great day dawned. Ena had prepared the dining room with a finicky thoroughness. The tables were all pushed together to make a square, and the best tablecloth was produced from some hidden store. Ena had even found ten sets of chopsticks and set them on the table under the mistaken impression that they were the traditional implements for curry eating. She also thoughtfully provided spoons and forks for the less culturally aware. She even put flowers in the centre of the table, the 'get well soon' message in the middle of them betraying their origins. Ena had also gone to the trouble of writing the doctors' names on little cards, and had made sure that there was an even mix of the warring factions. She had run out of these cards by the time she got to the Pharaoh, and he had a bigger card with 'FAIRO' on one side and 'Pathology Request' on the other. Ena summoned the doctors to their places wearing a short tight-fitting blue crimplene dress and a little frilly-edged white pinafore. She wore even more lipstick and mascara than usual. The doctors filed in and found their place settings. Some tried to swap so that they would be next to an ally, but Ena was having none of it: 'You stay where you're put, this is Madge and mine's treat and you'll do it wor way or there's no dinner for ye, right?'

Sheepishly the doctors bowed to this superior force, sat down and tried to make the best of it.

Resplendent in a large chef's hat and, for once, a clean white starched smock, Madge strutted into the room bearing a tray of various side dishes – cucumber raita, vegetable curry and a spinach bhaji, ground coconut, raisins and a large jar of pickled eggs. The latter dish is a strange Northern delicacy; usually consumed with copious quantities of Newcastle brown ale, a heavy deep brown beer known locally at that time as 'Journey into Space.' The beer is required to wash away the disgusting bitter vinegar taste. As a guide to the uninitiated, the nearest experience I can think of to eating a pickled egg is probably chewing a freshly painted old tennis ball. Madge thought they were so disgusting that the foreign doctors would be sure to love them. Ena brought in a large salver covered in steaming speckled pilau rice, and gingerly pushed it to the centre of the table, simultaneously exposing a large area of heavily veined white thigh and a set of suspenders of the kind usually only seen in Sunday newspaper adverts. Freddie's hand approached the forbidden zone and Ena automatically brushed it away as if shooing an annoying little fly. Then came Madge struggling with a large black Shakespearean cauldron three-quarters full of a powerful smelling, bubbling, lumpy brown mixture which she triumphantly placed on the table. She stood short and squat, with her ample bosom stuck out, challenging the assembled company to share her culinary achievement.

'Right lads, this is Madge's special lamb curry.' She half bowed and flourished her chef's hat like a medieval courtier, 'Get yer gobs roond that little lot and a diven't want any moanin'.'

Ena and Madge set about helping to dispense generous helpings all round, and then retired to one side of the room to await the unstinting praise that would surely follow. The luckless smiling Pharaoh was the first to try a large undiluted mouthful of the dark dripping meat. He chewed and swallowed it quickly, gesturing at Madge and Ena with an anglicised thumbs-up sign, but at that moment a change came over him. His normally dark, swarthy complexion suddenly changed to the same colour as the nicotine-stained white wallpaper, then there was another chameleon-like change to a deep bluish-green hue, and within a few more seconds his whole face became a sort of reddish black. Everyone in the room was transfixed by this *son et lumière* virtuoso performance. Suddenly a deep, choking, agonised Egyptian oath escaped his lips and echoed eerily around the room. He shot bolt upright, knocking his chair over in the process, clutched his throat and ran, wild-eyed, from the room.

This had a somewhat unnerving effect on the spectators. Complete silence engulfed the table, fatty brown lumps were pushed gingerly around plates, lumps were dissected into tiny pieces smothered in rice and chewed with extreme nervous deliberation while anxiously watching the others for signs of acute toxicity. In fact, after the first two or three mouthfuls the pain went, to be replaced by a buzzing numb feeling that extended from the forehead to the Adam's apple. The experience even became pleasurable in a masochistic sort of way. Madge, somewhat disconcerted by the Pharaoh's exit, ventured a prompt.

'Well, worra ye think then?'

Those who could speak were mainly from Southern India, used to fearsomely hot curries.

'Bit much chilli, Madge, but not bad for a memsahib.' Others nodded as best they could, and gradually the curry and the side dishes began to disappear, conversation resumed, and even became animated, and sworn enemies laughed together. Briefly the mess was a happy place. After a while Madge voiced the anxiety of the others: 'Where's that fond fool the Pharaoh, aah think a bit must've gone doon the wrang way if ye ask me. Ena be a gud lass an gan and luk fer him, make sure he's alreet.'

Ena found him some time later clutching the children's drinking fountain in the hospital car park, with a deathly pale complexion, streaming eyes and completely incapable of speech. She led him back to his room like a sick animal and stayed with him for some time. He never ate in the mess again, surviving on a diet of Egyptian biscuits sent from home, and salami sausage and rye bread from the grocer over the road, but Ena went to his room a lot after that day, her suspendered thighs offering him some solace in a lonely country.

Not long afterwards a curry house opened opposite the hospital, ambitiously called 'The Gourmet.' This was too much for the Geordie tongue, and it was soon universally known as 'The Gummit.' Once a week the doctors clubbed together and enjoyed a glutinous take-away evening. Madge was never called upon to perform again, but was held in increased respect by the entire mess from the time of that memorable meal.

As for the Pharaoh, with Ena's help he struggled through the last few months of his attachment, doctors and nurses alike ensuring that as far as possible he was kept away from any patients, especially sick ones. He gave up his English lessons, but took up painting, for which he had quite a talent. Just before he left, he presented the mess with a large canvas of the famous curry evening. He called it 'The Last Supper.'

Chapter 23

Smallpox on a passenger liner

Darwin in North Australia is a strange place, and in 1971 its charms were certainly limited. There is a feeling of isolation about this town that is confirmed by a look at the map. The most exciting shop was Woolworth's, and the sidewalks were still reminiscent more of Tombstone than of a modern city. A year later a terrible typhoon did untold damage, but here on Christmas Eve a chain of events, much less dramatic but of more personal significance, was about to unfold. I was the senior surgeon on the liner *Orcades*, and she had been delayed because of electrical trouble in the boiler room. Twelve hours in Darwin is a long time, and three days seemed like a lifetime. A kind of torpid languor had engulfed passengers and crew alike. Just how many times can you see Robert Shaw doing a pretty lacklustre impression of Custer of the West and stare at the range of insect repellents and rat poisons which seemed to be Woolworth's main stock? Still, we cleared them out of fairy lights and artificial snow, but Christmassy it wasn't. A few of the crew dressed up in coats, scarves and gloves and went carol singing. They carried lanterns and sang about gathering winter fuel and being in the deep midwinter as the temperature hovered around 100 degrees in the shade. Mad dogs and Englishmen.

Early on Christmas morning the phone rang. Could I come and look at someone with a weird rash? The patient was a Goanese crew member, one of a batch of 20 or so who had been flown into Singapore around five days ago to relieve others due leave. The young man's symptoms were spots and a slight fever. The spots were on his arms and chest, raised from the surface of the skin, with a central dimple, and in medical jargon 'umbilicated.'

All the internal red lights went on at once. The differential diagnosis was both mundane and terrifying. Chickenpox was favourite, followed by insect bites, or a kind of skin infection commonly called impetigo – but, and it was a very big but, the spots themselves matched the classic textbook description of smallpox. Was there smallpox where he came from? Goa, now an international package holiday destination, was then a small province on the west coast of mainland India, notable for its Catholic religion and its beautiful but very poor populace. P&O had a longstanding arrangement with Goanese employment organisations, and had been recruiting inexpensive male crew for several decades. Their religion and their temperament made them eminently suitable for service on big white liners as waiters, cabin servants and cooks. However, they were living in Third World conditions at home, and several diseases now extinct in more developed countries were still endemic in their home environment. The $64,000 question was whether smallpox was one of these diseases.

It was still very early in the morning, about 7 a.m., and at last the ship was fixed and just setting out on its way to a stop at a top tourist spot on the Great Barrier Reef, Hayman Island. This was a good two days' sail away. Now smallpox anywhere is a terror, but on a passenger liner it is a disaster of Hollywood proportions. Smallpox is one of the most infectious diseases that we know of, and it also has a truly frightening mortality rate, ranging from nearly 100% to 20–30% at best, depending on the strain of the virus and the susceptibility of the community affected. In recent years we have become accustomed to thinking of it as a weapon of terrorism, since the disease itself was wiped out by the WHO's vaccination pro-gramme, the last non-laboratory case occurring in the early 1980s. Even at the time about which I am writing it was rare, and was confined to poor populations in hot countries. Doctors who had been trained in the UK had no actual experience of the illness – their knowledge was all theoretical and historical. Luckily there were still doctors who did have experience. As a senior officer I had my own table in the restaurant with eight allotted passengers, one of whom was a retired colonial medical officer, last stationed in Burma and now on his way home to England for the last time. He came to the surgery without demur, the old medical antennae sensing a crisis and a chance to be useful. He was thorough and professional. We went into my office and he shook his head gravely. 'That's variola (the Latin name for smallpox) or I'm a Dutchman. Probably variola minor, you know it's a slightly attenuated version but still nasty, and can sometimes revert back to the real McCoy. I am bl**** glad I'm not in your shoes – and it's Christmas, too.' I can still remember that sinking feeling.

Dominico needed isolating. We were lucky in that respect, as the ship's hospital was situated over the propeller at C deck aft. There was a small self-contained room there designed for just this purpose, known as the brig, as it also doubled as a cell should the need arise to restrain an aggressive crew member or passenger. I tried to explain to Dominico why this was being done. He became distressed, and although his English was poor it was clear that he disagreed with the diagnosis, and he had to be strong-armed into the brig, but doctor–patient relationships were not the number one priority in this situation. That priority was telling the Captain what we were facing. The Australians were already renowned for being the fussiest nation on earth when it came to health matters on ships, so they were not going to take kindly to this news, and neither was the Captain. I said I was sorry to bother him at this hour, he told me to get on with it, and I suggested that he should pour himself a gin first. He said he never drank at this time of day and no news could be that bad. I said that we had a case of smallpox on board, and he asked if I would like a gin, too.

The Captain stared at me, asked me how sure I was, and I told him about the experienced second opinion. We could be wrong, but the odds and the seriousness were such that we had to treat the risk as real. He gulped a large gin down in one and summoned the staff captain, the chief officer and the purser. The chief engineer was still nursing his boilers back to rude health. It was the gloomiest senior officer call I ever attended. This disease killed people, and it could, given half a chance, kill lots of people, and senior ship's officers were not immune. I was asked for my recommendations. It sounds awful but I was starting to enjoy this situation in a vicarious sort of way. Here I was, 25 years old and a senior surgeon, giving my advice to very experienced men, mostly in their late forties or early fifties. It was a big change from being a houseman, where I was used to being only one up from the hospital cat, and that was only when there were no mice around.

The staff captain wondered what we should tell the passengers and when, and the purser wondered whether we should shut the restaurant and feed everyone sandwiches. The Captain wondered to himself whether this would be his last voyage. We concocted a short note to be delivered to all passengers, which stated that we had a case of smallpox on board, but that it was mild and the patient had been isolated. Then we radioed the Darwin Port Health Authority, who said that we could not go back, and suggested that we should talk to the authorities in Brisbane. Eventually the Captain spoke briefly, and I was handed the radio to talk to the Australian Chief Medical Officer. He was an irritable-sounding man with no discernible sense of humour, not that the situation was funny. He insisted that everyone on board should be inspected 24-hourly, but 12-hourly within 48 hours of landfall and, yes, everyone on board without a valid certificate must be vaccinated, no excuses tolerated. He did give the impression that he was as certain as he could be that our diagnosis was wrong and this was probably a storm in a teacup and of course it was only chickenpox in an Asian man. We were to move out of Australian Territorial Waters and make our way to Brisbane for further instructions. The Great Barrier Reef stop was summarily cancelled.

The Chief Medical Officer had insisted that only the ship's doctors could do the inspections, but had agreed that the nurses could help with the vaccinations. There were only two doctors and two nurses, plus Ron the former naval dispenser, who counted as a nurse as far as I was concerned. Fortunately there was already an established inspection routine before docking in Australian ports. The port health authority ruled that any ship from a non-Australian port must undergo a full smallpox inspection before being allowed to dock, so that we were used to doing such inspections before docking in Fremantle on the journey over from South Africa, and recently we had just inspected the passengers before docking in Darwin on our way down from Singapore. So there was an established routine, and even an expectation of this among both the passengers and the crew, but doing it for four days, twice a day for the last two days was going to severely tax everyone's patience, and would finally put to the test the much vaunted stamina of two young doctors.

The purser got all the crew together and told them the situation. The Goanese crew members took it especially badly, perceiving this event as a form of victimisation, and a slur on their good name and hygiene, and all were convinced that it was chickenpox misdiagnosed by a sybaritic doctor who was wet behind the ears and just out of Western medical school. To be honest, Martin, the assistant surgeon, and I were beset by doubt ourselves. In the 12 hours since diagnosis, Dominico appeared no worse physically, although emotionally he was far from chipper, not helped by our hospital attendant's grim jibes that he could have anything to eat that he wanted, so long as it was flat and could be pushed under the door. By the time this had been laboriously translated by the chief pantryman it had lost any intrinsic humour, and caused loud sobs and wails of anguish. We were now doing our best to barrier nurse Dominico, but the green outfits (which were full of holes due to the sheer age of the gowns) and the rather full dental-type face masks did nothing to make the poor soul feel cared for.

There was pressure from many passengers to have an explanatory meeting, as the note that we had issued, while not exactly causing panic, had generated much anxiety. Everyone was summoned to the main ballroom and the staff captain did his best, but the mood was not that of the Blitz – it was more like that which prevailed just before the storming of the Bastille. In view of this similarity, the purser's decision to let the passengers eat even more cake seemed an appropriate one. Each passenger was to be given a goodie pack/extra Christmas present by way of compensation for the restrictions that were about to be imposed.

Medically we decided to combine the first inspection with the mass vaccination, and we did the crew first – to get our hand in, as it were. We decided to vaccinate all of the Goanese crew regardless of what was stated on their smallpox certificate. This was because to a man they were all notorious needle haters and it was well known that most of the certificates were forged (this was a cottage industry in Goa). Vaccination was undertaken by placing a drop of serum on the skin, scratching two parallel lines at right angles to each other, and rubbing the serum into the scratches with a needle. It was not a painful procedure, but the reaction of many would belie that fact. We brooked no excuses, however elaborate. The purser also had a bright idea for giving the passengers some backbone. He played Verdi's Grand March from *Aida* at high volume from the ballroom speakers, and such stirring music did have a profound morale-boosting effect. We got to bed in the early hours and dreamt of spots, arms and pyramids. *Orcades* steamed, all boilers working now, up and round the North Australian coast. Dominico cried himself into a fitful sleep, robotically fiddling with his rosary, and a few more spots appeared just to keep the tension up.

The next morning we inspected the newly arrived Goanese with a fine-tooth comb. We made them strip to the buff and we then examined them all over, but luck was with us, as no one else had any spots. This inspection was much more thorough than that which we accorded the rest of the ship's complement. The accepted wisdom was that smallpox was a centri-fugal illness whereas chickenpox was a centripetal one. This translated into the fact that the easy way to inspect for smallpox was to examine the forearms and face, as these were the most likely places for the spots to first appear. Chickenpox mainly starts on the trunk. However, like everything in medicine, this is a guide, not a certainty. It also meant that we did not need to insist on passengers shuffling through disrobed, which was likely to start a riot, or at least uncontrollable giggling.

The mechanics of the passenger inspection were complex. The ballroom on A deck was assigned for the purpose. We two ship's doctors were stationed towards one end on either side, and the passengers were divided into two rows that shuffled down towards us, rolling up their sleeves as they came. Each doctor was assigned a woman assistant purser to check the passenger list and see that the names were ticked off properly. Meanwhile male assistant pursers were responsible for general policing of the lines and seeking out recalcitrants. For the inspectors it was tedious work. The repartee about seeing spots, spotty Muldoon, big pox not smallpox, etc. soon palled. Many passengers tried to eke out bits of information on how many fresh cases there were, and were palpably disbelieving when told that there was still only one. The rumour machine already had us treating dozens in a secret location somewhere in the crew quarters. Being asked when the proper doctors were going to be flown in was a particularly irritating common refrain. Other than arms and faces the view was blue – just sea and lots of it. So for four days until Brisbane, twice daily for the last two days, this inspection ritual continued.

Dominico never became really ill, but by the time we were approaching Brisbane Harbour he had an impressive array of spots at all stages of development. We were really lucky in that no one else had developed the disease, and our strategies had seemed to be effective. There was a cautious optimism in the air. However, the Australian Port Health Authority did not share this feeling. They were taking no chances, and we were not even allowed into the harbour, but were told to anchor outside. We were also instructed to fly two yellow flags. Normally only one yellow flag was flown prior to being cleared by the port health authority. Two yellow flags signified that we were a dangerous pariah. Fortunately it was a calm blue day, and the passengers got word that the proper doctors were coming, so a large gathering appeared at the railings to watch for their arrival. After what seemed like an age, a disappointingly ordinary little launch pootled its way out to the ship. We were waiting at the main passenger door, and the launch gangway was lowered. Three spacemen appeared wearing full-protection barrier suits with proper visors, white gloves and white wellington boots. The lead spaceman spoke to me. I couldn't understand anything he said, as it was all muffled by the visor and was probably in a strong Australian accent to boot, so I nodded, made a traditional thumbs-up gesture and led them to the hospital anyway. Dominico was beside himself with terror as this group entered the claustrophobic and dingy little brig. The last of the spacemen unpacked what seemed like a large piece of clingfilm and wrapped poor Dominico in it. He stuck a snorkel-like thing in his mouth and continued wrapping. A fourth spaceman appeared in the doorway, with light glowing from his visor and pushing a shiny hospital trolley – it really was surreal. Dominico was trussed like a cooked chicken, unceremoniously grabbed and dumped on the trolley, and then whisked away, his breathing tube poking through the wrapping. He looked like an insect chrysalis. We never saw him again. The spacemen left quite unceremoniously, and did not even bother to try to talk again to what was obviously to them a lower life form.

The passengers shuffled away disconsolately, obviously disappointed at the rather poor show. Nothing happened for hours, while we remained bobbing somewhat nauseously at anchor, with the fleshpots of Brisbane tantalisingly visible. Eventually we received a radio communication from the port health authority. We could lower one yellow flag and proceed to a berth, but no one was to disembark until we received further instruction and, almost as an afterthought, smallpox inspections were to continue 12-hourly until further notice. There was mutiny afoot – Brisbane was just too near for this forced incarceration to be tolerated for long. Passengers besieged the ship's bureau, voices were raised, the masters at arms (ship's policemen) took up stations, and the staff captain and purser fretted over strategies to defuse the tension, neither of them being able to think of anything very useful. The Captain got on the radio to P&O head office, known as 'The Company', and told them that they must do something and soon. If strings needed pulling, well pull them now, or he would not be responsible for the consequences, which looked like an imminent break-down in civil order on the ship. It was round about this time that the chief pantryman, leader of the Goanese community, tapped me on the shoulder. 'Please come to the crew quarters', he said, 'Another crew member is sick and has spots.' My legs momentarily went a bit funny and a strange fizzing feeling engulfed my head – my mouth really did go dry. The Greek word 'hubris' echoed round my brain. The smell of curry permeated the whole dingy warren that was the Goanese quarters, none of the light bulbs appeared to emit more than 20 watts, and the overall impression was of a brown colour. This was not dirt – it was style. The patient was cowering in the darkest part of a gloomy cabin, and we could not see if he was wearing a shirt let alone if he had spots. Someone shone a powerful torch and he peeled off his shirt very reluctantly to reveal a panorama of spots, but my spirits soared – they were the wrong sort of spots. Joy! This chap had urticaria, and to my knowledge smallpox did not feature in the list of possible causes.

At last the port health authority came up with a ruling. All disembarking passengers should be inspected one last time and then allowed to leave, on the condition that they reported to the port health authority every 24 hours for a further three days. All other passengers and crew were confined to the ship. We were to continue inspections until we reached Sydney, three days' sailing away, and if there were still no more cases of smallpox we would be declared infection free. This was just enough to stop a riot, and by this time the ship's entertainment staff were organising all manner of activities, including such cruising staples as frog racing, deck tennis contests and a passenger-based music hall. The spirit of the Blitz did at last materialise and the renowned wry Aussie humour reasserted itself, often by means of inordinate consumption of 'tinnies' in the Ocean Bar.

Although we made several enquiries, Brisbane Port Health Authority never confirmed Dominico's condition as smallpox, but they never said it wasn't either. I remain convinced that we saw the last case of smallpox on a passenger liner.

Chapter 24

A big electrician, a bigger shock and the biggest ship

In 1971 I was the senior surgeon on the liner *Orcades*. It was 'coming home from Australia' time. Perth is a pretty city, but its port, Fremantle, is not. So there was little regret on our departure as we set off across the wide expanse of the Indian Ocean, our next landfall, Durban, being five full sailing days away, with no land in sight at all until then. It was the longest single stretch *Orcades* ever sailed. However, this was puny compared with the route currently being taken by the ship that we were soon to meet.

Twenty-four hours out of Fremantle in the middle of the night there was a summons to the radio room for an urgent medical consultation with an unnamed ship's master. I was handed the chunky radio telephone – the reception, as ever, was poor, with much crackling and hissing – and a nervous voice spoke rapidly in poor English with a strong Scandinavian accent. The drift was that there had been an accident and that a senior crew member was seriously injured, but how seriously? It was a bad line and the master, for it was he on the phone, repeated the story. While his chief electrician had been repairing electrical wiring on top of one of the ship's boilers, he had received a severe shock (the ship worked on 480 volts) and had been catapulted backwards and fallen at least 20 feet. He was still alive, but the Captain feared he was dying, and needed more assistance than he and his crew could provide.

A brief diversion into the ethics of this particular doctor–patient relationship may illuminate this situation. The company, P&O, did not mind me dispensing medical advice to all and sundry, but they did mind if doing so altered the ship's itinerary, because that cost money. So the onus was on the surgeon to deal with medical matters there and then with whatever advice seemed useful, and to avoid a rendezvous at any cost unless it really was a matter of life and death, and even then you had to be as sure as possible that the patient would live with your ministrations and die without them. If they were going to die anyway, that was just hard luck. This meant becoming a medical interrogator – gleaning as many facts as possible in order to get as clear a risk–benefit profile as possible. The final decision was made by the Captain, and he would usually consult with the company.

It quickly became apparent that the electrician was in a lot of pain, and the master needed advice on the appropriate dose and frequency of morphine that the ship was carrying in its medical supplies. The nature of the pain suggested chest wall injuries, front and back, and possible vertebral damage in the lower thoracic and upper lumbar region. For-tunately there appeared to be no sign of paralysis, so for the moment it did not seem that the spinal cord had been damaged, although the master knew that if there was a fractured vertebra, injudicious movement could be disastrous. The two most pressing concerns were that the man was peeing blood and getting paler and more ill by the hour. This strongly suggested internal injury to at least one kidney, and possible internal bleeding due to injury to other organs, such as the liver or spleen. If, as seemed likely, he had several fractured ribs, the displaced jagged ends could easily spear such organs, with very unpleasant consequences, both for him and for me. He was clearly in deep trouble, but could we help him?

Time to ask the Captain, who was not best pleased at being woken in the middle of the night, as he was well past 50. He was also perturbed – this was a bad time to have to consider slowing down, as there was a whole array of deadlines ahead, and with it being such a long crossing, fuel as well as being costly was in limited supply. Stopping and restarting engines apparently used up a disproportionate amount of the stuff. However, he was a good man with a humanitarian soul, and he wanted to do what was right, but he had to be sure. I was to report back after the next medical bulletin, but in the meantime the officer of the watch was to ascertain the speed and direction of the other ship and to work out the most efficient course needed to converge, with the implicit understanding that if any major alteration of course was needed, this was to be undertaken by the other ship.

The two hours passed in no time, and the report indicated that the man's condition was probably worsening. His blood pressure seemed to be slipping downwards as his pulse increased – a bad combination and a further indication of likely internal bleeding. He probably needed surgery, he would soon definitely need blood, and both ships were a minimum of two days from land in any direction. There is a commonly held myth that anything serious that goes wrong on a ship can be rectified by dispatching a helicopter. This is rubbish now and it was certainly rubbish in 1972. The range for a helicopter is quite small, and with only two to three hours of sailing most ships were out of range unless they were hugging the coast. We were by now nearly 48 hours away from Australia, way out of range of any such aid. In the meantime the company had made it plain to our Captain that there was to be no turning back as part of any equation. He told me this as he weighed the options. He appreciated that it was my medical recommendation that the electrician should be taken on board to give him at least a fighting chance. We could probably transfuse him and if the need was desperate even operate, as without such intervention he was likely to die within the next day or so.

We had found out the name of the ship – she was called the *Berge Istra*, but our Lloyds list did not have any information on her, presumably because she was too new. We also knew her course now. She was on what was termed 'a grand circle' from Buenos Aires to Yokohama, an enormous distance to cover without stopping (you need to look at a globe to visualise where we were intersecting). Her master had agreed to alter course, and ours had been given permission to stop for as short a period as possible to take the ill man on board. We were going to meet in about 12 hours. We all hoped, but for many different reasons, that it would not be too late.

The Captain invited me to the bridge to get the first glimpse of the *Berge Istra*. The recent medical reports on the electrician were worrying, but he was still alive. At last the bosun shouted and pointed to a blip on the radar, and we stared at it. The Captain squinted. 'That's a flaming big blip!' he exclaimed, and looked with binoculars at the horizon, then shook his head in disbelief as he handed them to me. 'The size of her, surgeon, just look at the size of her!' She was a monster, a huge long green monster. As she came alongside us, our relative sizes became plain. We were a big passenger ship – 28,000 tons give or take – but we could have been a lifeboat for this one. It transpired that at that time she was the biggest ship on the planet. Alongside, but at some distance, there was a big swell running, and we were still about a quarter of a mile away but as close as both Captains dared to approach. The *Berge Istra* was a colossal multi-purpose carrier and brand spanking new, her very size calming the sea between the two vessels. She was twin-funnelled, positioned as far aft as possible behind the slab-like bridge and living quarters. In front of the quarters was a huge stretch of deck with at least nine large battened-down hatches. Emblazoned in large white letters against the green sides was the inscription, *Bergesen D.Y. Tankers*. I knew I should go over to her to supervise the transfer of the injured man, but our Captain refused to let me go. He said it was too risky and he couldn't afford to lose a surgeon, but I suspected it was because it would take too much time. It was a big disappointment. The passengers were all crowding the upper decks to marvel at this leviathan and watch the show, and the word was out that we were picking up a severely injured sailor. It was too great a distance to attach a line between the two ships, but the crew of the *Berge Istra* were great professionals. Within an amazingly short time they had lowered a tiny-looking red lifeboat, strapped the injured man into a wrap-around stretcher (named after its designer, Anderson), and secured him as tightly as possible. The lifeboat bobbed across in double-quick time. We had opened the aft door, to be nearer the hospital, and the lifeboat docked. Seven large sailors then quickly but gently unloaded their comrade. They shook hands, accepted a crate of whisky with our Captain's compliments, and were off again. The whole transfer took less than 20 minutes. Both ships restarted their engines, hooted at each other, the passengers cheered and the amazingly small crew of the *Berge Istra* waved back, and we went our separate ways, but the memory of that great green beauty is still vivid over 30 years later.

We had our patient on board and had carried him to the hospital when the first problem presented itself. He, like his ship, was huge. So huge in fact that he was too long for our hospital beds – he was 6 feet 8 inches tall. We made him comfortable on one bed while the ship's carpenter sawed off the foot of the other bed. The patient was as pale as a ghost but was able to talk, and his English was good although his nationality was Swedish. His name was Hans and he was very poorly. His pulse was thin and fast, his blood pressure was low and he was in agony every time he urinated because of blood clots in the urine. On closer examination it seemed that a lower left rib had ripped into the left kidney. More ominously it looked as if he had a ruptured spleen, too. His abdomen was tense and exquisitely tender, and the muscle hardened on light touch. This was probably due to blood in the peritoneal cavity, but it could indicate a ruptured bowel. If that was the case he was definitely a goner.

All in all, his chances of reaching Durban did not look too bright, and the first priority was to give him some blood and to control his pain as much as possible. This was not easy at this time on a passenger liner, as we could not carry stores of blood, and the blood substitutes available then were not much good. The cross-matching was primitive, done with a series of blotting papers, a methodology devised by a Norwegian, which did in the end save a Swede from a Norwegian ship. There was a little book of blood groups of crew who were prepared to donate blood in an emergency. I cross-matched Hans, and again luck was not on his side. It was not on Colin's side either. Colin was the chief officer, and the only person listed who was AB+ like Hans. He was a big florid man, but he was a lot less florid by the time we got to Durban. In fact when I asked him to come to the hospital and it gradually became clear to him that he was the only person who stood between this huge Swede and eternity, all the colour drained out of his cheeks and his normal ebullient expansiveness evaporated, but he knew his duty. We hitched Colin up to the bottle, with those old red rubber tubes now long since replaced by transparent plastic, and took a pint off him, which we gave straight to Hans. For such a big man it was just a drop in a bucket, but we gave him some reconstituted plasma to bulk it out, too. After a few hours the clot colic began to ease and his urine began to clear, so at least the kidney bleeding was stopping, but what about the spleen?

Operating on a passenger liner at this time was very much a last resort. Putting people to sleep is easy (well, in our case, easy-ish). The trick is waking them up again and not gassing yourself with the ether in the process. This meant that our strategy had to be to avoid operation if humanly possible, and to try to keep poor Hans alive for the three more days it would take to reach Durban, but if an operation was his only chance . . . I got the surgical textbook out again. Human beings, unlike cars or washing machines, do not come with detailed repair manuals, more's the pity. The nearest we had then were surgical and anatomical textbooks. I read the section on spleens – 'Cut along dotted line A, tie off B, dissect out C, etc.' – poor Hans, he hadn't got a hope. An appendix I could just about manage, but a splenectomy – no way. I phoned Colin again and asked him how he was feeling. He got the drift immediately – you didn't need a videophone to visualise his expression. He bravely 'volunteered' to donate another pint. I can't take all of the credit for his noble self-sacrifice. It was really down to Brenda, our senior nurse, who at this time was having a brief but extremely physical relationship with the aforesaid Colin. That was if the noises emanating from her cabin late at night were to be taken at face value. I have reason to believe that in order to stiffen (if that is the right word) Colin's shaky resolve the spirit of Lycistrita was invoked.

After the second pint Hans really did start to improve. His blood pressure stabilised, his pulse rate at last started to drop below 100, his temperature was down and, perhaps most importantly, he started to think he might make it. He began talking, and it turned out that he was born in Gothenburg, but his current domicile was an address in the

Scotty Road, Liverpool, where he was ensconced with a young Scouse woman. He had met the Beatles, been regularly to the Cavern Club, and had had a few drinks with John Lennon. He had started his career at the age of 17, apprenticed to the Blue Funnel line which was based in Liverpool, known after its founder as 'Alfred Holt's Navy', and got this plum job on the maiden voyage of the *Berge Istra*, which was owned by a Norwegian shipping magnate. The *Istra* was to be part of a fleet of huge carriers with the prefix *Berge*. One reason for getting the job was his proficiency in languages – he spoke at least seven, even if his English was flavoured by a not unattractive mix of Swedish and Liverpudlian dialect. In no time he was chatting up Brenda, a fact that didn't go unnoticed by the increasingly anaemic Colin, but neither of the men was really feeling up to any action – in any case it was just fun and probably aided the healing.

With 24 hours to go, Hans' condition took a turn for the worse, probably because he was trying to do too much and shuffled off to the loo by himself rather than suffer the indignity and humiliation of the bedpan. The ship rolled a little, he slipped and the bleeding started again. I really did think we were going to have to operate this time. We gave him a large dose of morphine and a sedative to knock him out, and those of a religious persuasion prayed for him, especially Colin. With 12 hours to go, and Hans showing slow but definite deterioration, could Colin manage just a further half pint? He did. I don't know if he will be rewarded in heaven, but after his recovery a week or so later he was certainly rewarded on this earth according to reports. That was enough – Hans made it to Durban, where the ambulance and surgical team were waiting. He was in fact even more damaged than we had thought. Both kidneys were injured, his liver capsule was torn and oozing internally, and yes – the spleen was ruptured. I believe they aspirated at least four pints from his peritoneal cavity, two and a half of which had belonged to Colin. His spleen was removed together with a third of his left kidney, and he was transfused with a further six pints of blood, but he made it, and within two months was back in Liverpool.

For a few years he sent me Christmas cards with little snippets about his life – and yes, he was back on the *Berge Istra*. By this time I was a family doctor, and as I listened to the radio one morning while doing my visits, there was a news bulletin reporting the tragic loss of one of the biggest ships in the world – you guessed it, the *Berge Istra*. She had gone down with the loss of all hands in the South China Sea. I stopped the car and couldn't continue for some time. I just knew that Hans had not cheated death twice. It later transpired that the cause was probably inadequate clearing of the holds of inflammable gases before loading a full cargo of iron ore in Japan. There was an explosion that ruptured the hull, and the ship had sunk like a stone. At Lloyds of London they rang the Lutine Bell.

Chapter 25

A terrible illness

Passenger ships are fairly unhealthy places. Apart from the obvious sea sickness, minor ailments are common. The newest liners are often swept by gastrointestinal viruses despite stringent hygiene regulations, and *Orcades*, one of the old school, had her own special variety of a debilitating wheezy flu-like illness that many passengers contracted after a few days on board. We never did any bacteriological or viral studies, but I suspect that some evil bug lived in the air-conditioning system. On longer voyages it was not uncommon for up to half of the passengers to be affected at some time or other. This ensured that a steady stream of not very ill passengers came to the surgery each day – 40 was not an unusual figure, and at $5 a time in 1970 and with profit on antibiotics and X-rays the income became considerable. A few passengers developed quite severe chest infections and needed cabin or hospital care with high doses of antibiotics. During a long cruise it was not unusual to have four or five people in hospital at any one time. Legionnaire's disease had not been discovered then, but I sometimes wonder if some of the more severe illnesses were caused by a similar organism, perhaps not as virulent as it now appears to be. Certainly the conditions for spread with the old-fashioned, air-blown punkahs were ideal. Mild gastric upsets were also common, and small outbreaks of gastroenteritis were not infrequent. The P&O surgeons didn't complain. It was all good for business, and I suspect that it still is.

Occasionally passengers came on board with severe illness. The Pillings were the worst. They had taken the unusual step of booking for the whole voyage – Southampton to Southampton – which would take a period of over five months. Amazingly, as it turned out, they didn't come to my attention until just after the start of the first cruise from Sydney, some six weeks into the voyage. Cecil, the purser, approached me in the surgery one morning. 'Surgeon', he was always very formal, 'I am very worried about the passengers Mr and Mrs Pilling in cabin B12. Something is very wrong. Mr Pilling has insisted that no one enters the cabin at all and has booked for the whole voyage. All his food is placed outside at mealtimes and he insists on changing the linen himself. The sheets are in a disgusting state, excreta everywhere, and the cabin is beginning to smell terribly.' It sounded very odd.

'What explanation does Mr Pilling give?'

'Ah, that's just it. He doesn't give any. He won't tell me anything, though I have pressed him, he refuses all help and he won't let me see his wife. My staff and I now feel that in the interests of general health we must insist on access to the cabin.'

Cecil and I went to the Captain, Cecil repeated the story and I asked the Captain to give me permission to force entry if absolutely necessary. 'What do you think is wrong, doctor?', he asked.

'You know, sir, I just don't have the faintest idea, though it sounds as if Mrs Pilling is terminally ill, but why he doesn't want anyone to see her is a mystery.'

The senior nurse and I knocked at the door of cabin B12. There was no reply, but there was a very strong smell of ill human being oozing out. We continued knocking, but still there was no response except for a sound of shuffling and barricading from within. We tried another gambit and walked along to the telephone exchange and rang the cabin from there. After a long time Mr Pilling answered. 'Hello, Mr Pilling, this is Dr Tate speaking, the ship's surgeon. I would like to offer my help and that of my staff. Please could I come to your cabin to talk it over?'

'Oh no, please no, doctor,' he was weeping, 'Please leave us alone.'

'I'm afraid I can't do that. The Captain has asked me to help you, by forcible entry if necessary. I don't want to do anything like that, so perhaps you would like to come to my surgery and tell me your wife's problem?' I could hear him sobbing. 'Mr Pilling, are you all right?'

'Yes, yes, doctor. All right, I will come now, but please don't let anyone in.'

Mr Pilling was a tall haggard man with a pale yellow, sickly complexion, aged about 65. He looked as if he hadn't shaved for at least three days. 'Sit down, please, and try to tell me what's wrong. You look at the end of your tether.' He buried his head in his hands, his whole body shook with despair and he wept some more. I put my hand on his shoulder and waited. Slowly he looked up. 'She's dying, doctor, but it's so slow and so horrible for her.' He stared in front of him.

'Has she got cancer?' I asked, trying to prompt him gently.

'Oh no, God no. That would be a kindness compared with this. She's got Huntington's chorea. Do you know about it?' Sadly I did.

Just to remind you, this is a ghastly inherited condition, first described in 1872 by the physician who gave it its name. It is a dominant gene with complete penetrance. This means that if a parent has the illness, there is a fifty-fifty chance of any child getting it. The illness develops in middle life and is steadily progressive, usually giving 15–20 years between onset and death. There is progressive mental deterioration associated with uncontrollable movements of the arms, legs, body and head, and there is no cure. In the moderate-sized market town where I became a GP we had three families with this dreadful gene, most of which were traced back to an amorous American serviceman.

'Yes, Mr Pilling, I do know about it. How long has she had it?'

'Fifteen years now, but it's near the end – that's why I brought her to sea. Do you understand?'

'Well, not really, tell me.'

'Well, she's so ashamed, she's so out of control she didn't want any of her friends to see her like this. She wanted to die away from them and she didn't want to go into a hospital, so I thought of taking her to sea on a long trip to die with a little dignity.' What a burden this man was carrying – it was impossible not to be almost overwhelmed by pity for him. He needed help and he knew it. He stared at me, wide-eyed and despairing.

'Please let me see her.' He made a decision.

'All right, all right, doctor, but only you and your nurse, no one else.'

I will never ever forget Cabin B12. He led Elizabeth the nurse and me inside. It was dark, all the portholes were shuttered and it was indescribably foetid. All the punkahs were turned off and it smelled very strongly of human waste and illness. As my eyes adjusted I saw on the bed a tiny skeletal lady continually writhing and twitching, her head moving constantly in a circular way. She recognised that I was not her husband, and recoiled from my presence like a frightened animal, whimpering pathetically. I moved a little closer, and she recoiled even more. I was at a loss to know what to do.

'Please let me help you, Mrs Pilling. I am a doctor. I may be able to lessen your suffering, and my nurses could help you and your husband a great deal.' She lay cowering and twitching on the bed, making movements of fending me off. She didn't reply, and there was no way of telling if she even understood me. I turned to her distraught husband. 'Please let me help her. I can sedate her and perhaps control the worst of some of the movements. The nurses can bath her and change the sheets.' In tears he agreed, nodding slowly. Like most of us in crisis he had wanted someone to take the decision for him, but his debt of honour was a considerable burden.

We did our best. A few drugs helped a little, particularly haloperidol, a well-known tranquilliser, which in small doses seemed to calm her, and she became slightly less fearful. The nurses cleaned her and the cabin. It was so painful for her to accept even this help that we kept our distance and visited only once a day. She never saw Matavi Bay in Tahiti, or heard the Fijian singers in Savu Savu, she didn't eat sukiyaki in Kobe or climb the peak in Hong Kong, and the greatest tragedy of all was that she lived to get back to Southampton.

Her daughter came aboard on a cold January morning to help them disembark, and she came to the hospital to thank the nurses and me for our help with her parents. As she talked her head moved slightly oddly, and she wouldn't meet my eye, but with an unsteady voice she said that her brother had committed suicide on hearing that his mother was returning. She thanked us for our kindness, but as she edged out of the cramped little hospital, she whispered 'I wish you hadn't been quite so kind, couldn't you have helped her die? I hope my own GP will help us all.' I hope he or she did.

Mickey

The outpatients department at Sunderland General Hospital in February 1969 was not the most fun-filled place to be. I don't need to describe it, as your imagination will do better – but I warn you, it was worse than that. I was the medical house officer drafted in to see the 'chronics.' These were the living dead, with advanced incurable illnesses for which medicine had no solution, and precious little comfort. As the most junior doctor in the hospital it was reasoned that I couldn't make them any worse and the cleverer doctors could be utilised on the newer patients who might just be more interesting, if no less curable. It was late in the afternoon, and I was subdued and a little cowed by the inevitability of it all. Remember I was only 22 and wanted to make a difference to people's suffering, but there didn't seem to be a way. Then I met Mickey.

He was a little man, maybe five foot nothing in his socks, with a chest like a barrel and a cherubic pink face with a smile to make your heart ache. He struggled into the cubicle ('room' would be too posh a word), gasping and clutching from one support to another. He was looking at me the whole time. He spoke in gasps that didn't seem to have any pauses between them. He had a chirrupy cheeky voice.

'Way Hinney, yor not oot of school surely, and yer the wrang colour fer this place. Ye need a coat of broon paint to be a doctor in Sunland.' I was on my feet trying to help him, but he shooed me away.

'Divvent need any help, be in me box soon enough, aal gerrall the help then, that's what the vicar says, but he's run off with the missus, so what would he kna, poor bugger.' He cackled wheezily, and sat with a rush, panting. I thought he was going to die there and then. I had no idea what I was supposed to do for Mickey, but this was not a unique feeling that afternoon. Mickey took a minute or so to get what little was left of his breath back, and I noticed that he was dressed in his Sunday best – collar, tie, starched shirt, full suit with waistcoat and silver fob chain and shiny black brogues. He looked as if he had just been redeemed from the pawnshop. He smelt overpoweringly of Vick and mothballs. *In extremis* there are standards to be maintained, and he was doing just that. Many of these attitudes died with his generation, and we are the poorer for it. But Mickey was the most fearlessly irreverent of men.

'Wey gan on, ask me how I am, do they teach you nuthin these days?'

'Er, how are you Mr Scott?' I obeyed, knowing I was outranked. Here was a dying man with experience of living – it was his show.

'Bloody knackered, aav nor enuff puff to blow oot a Lucifer.' He was triumphant to have got his opening gambit out with a finality that left few avenues to explore. I couldn't think of anything to say. I vaguely remembered that Lucifer was First World War slang for a match – some expressions linger in small communities.

'Lucifer, that's an odd word – match, isn't it?'

He broke into wheezy song, 'While you've a Lucifer to light your fag, smile boys that's the style, pack up your troubles in your old kit bag and smile smile smile.' He regrouped. 'Sang that at Dunkirk, drooned the noise of them Jerry Bastards in the Stukas. Me Da must have sung it too. Go to Wipers an put yer ear to the groond on Hill 16 and you might hear him singing it, a hundred feet doon.' I waited as he left no gap for me to respond. 'He was a miner, too, didn't live lang enough to die slow like me, boom and half of bloody Belgium on top of him. Aah were three months at the time.' I felt I ought to be a doctor, not a listener – always an unwise move – so I butted in.

'Do you need a new inhaler?'

He looked at me with a sort of head-shaking smile of despair for the ignorant.

'Look, yer daft happorth, yam tryin me best to tell you me story an your gannin on aboot puffers. Look, young doc, let's be clear. You can't cure me, aah doot you can help me, but the least ye can do is listen to me. Aave cum in me best canonicals, an it's norraneasy journey from Hetton. Give me some respect an I meet larn you summat.'

'Like what?' I said, a trifle crossly. It was late, I was nearly but not quite fed up, and Mickey was the last patient that afternoon.

'Aboot what it's like to be poorly. Ifn yer gannin to be any gud you've gorra understand what yer patients are gannin thru. De yees kna with the help of me missus, she didna run off with the vicar more's the pity, it took we nearly an hour just to get togged up to gan oot. We had to keep stoppin just to get breath. She had to put me troosers on us for God's sake. You imagine that, young un.' I didn't want to. I was unsure where this was leading, but I have always liked stories, and it seemed there were worse things to do than listen to Mickey's. I hadn't learned the trick of saying 'tell me more', but Mickey was going to tell me whether I liked it or not.

He looked into my eyes, right in deep, much deeper than any examiner I had met.

'Ye kna anythin aboot mining? Aave been doon Hetton pit since I were 14 with fower years off for gud behaviour scrappin with the Hun. An yer kna why aam like I am? It's cos aave got a bag of nutty slack in me chest.' I obviously looked confused.

'Nutty slack is them crappy little bits of coal they canna sell, so the pit owners generously hand it oot free to the workers, but if you've been doon lang enough you've already got a sackful in yer chest. Ifn yer set fire to us aad born for a week. You want ter see me spit.' It wasn't a question. Mickey took out a tightly wrapped little pot from an inside pocket. Sputum is not a glamorous human secretion, but this was different. The now unwrapped pot was opened to reveal a slimy translucent substance full of tiny black bits, and there could be no doubt that these little bits were indeed coal. An image of dissected black lungs shown in some long previous lecture came to mind. I knew now quite clearly what Mickey's lungs looked like from the inside. I felt a wave of sympathy, and he saw it.

'Aah don't want yer pity, but now ye kna what aam talkin aboot. There's none of yer medicines can get rid of that lot, ye kna the worst? Me missus is forever buyin washin pooder cos me hankies is allas (always) black with hoiking (coughing) this stuff into them.' He cackled again. I still didn't know if he wanted anything from me, but whatever it was, it wasn't sympathy.

'You a local lad?' I nodded. 'Like football?' I nodded again. 'Sunland?' I kept nodding. 'Charley Horley (Hurley)?' I smiled a big smile. Big Charlie was and remains my all-time Sunderland hero – a magnificent attacking centre half and a leader of men. I have his picture in my outside loo to this day. 'Dooin rotten at present mind you.' This was sadly true – nothing changes. 'Not won a game al year, ye kna my favourite? Captain Raich (Carter), Shack (Len Shackleton) was pretty canny, but the Captain, he was summit special. Aah canna gan anymore, didna miss a match for 30 yors, but aah haven't the puff now, aah canna gerrup the stairs. Shame, but at least I tell mesel there's nowt worth watchin. Dee yer want to listen?'

'Listen?'

'To me chest! They all want to listen, though Gawd knas what fower. Howay give us a hand wi me jacket and we'll find a gap fer yer tubes.' We did after a struggle. Mickey breathed and I listened. I expected wheezing and rattling but could not hear anything. I checked my stethoscope. Mickey grinned triumphantly. 'Nowt to hear, eh? One of them top clever clogs showed me off to the students once. Mister Taylor', he said in an exaggeratedly posh voice, 'has no sounds in his lungs because he has no air in them – you need air to produce the sound – he has silent lungs, a very advanced sign I am afraid.' He slipped back into deepest Wearside. 'That were five years ago, an he's deed, heart attack, an aam still battin. He said aah was a pink puffer. Aah thowt he was talkin aboot a train, but when he said the other sort was a blue bloater ah thowt he'd been doon to the fish quay. But ye kna, a couple of me mates were big an blue all ower, they're in their boxes noo.' Mickey was referring to the traditional description of the two types of respiratory failure, usually seen in miners. Skinny small gasping men who stayed pink to the end, and their friends who developed heart strain and then heart failure, known by the Latin name of cor pulmonale. They filled up with fluid and were cyanosed all of the time because not enough oxygen got into their bloodstream to make it the usual red colour. I began to help him get his jacket back on, and mentioned the possibility of a flu injection.

'Hadaway there's na point, de ye think ah want to keep living like this? Aah want the reaper to come, sooner the better if ye ask me. Protect us from flu!! It would be a god's blessing to get a quick vicious one kidda. The day I have one of them jabs will be the day I snuff it.' Prophetic, as it turned out. 'I betta be away noo, divvent want to miss the bus and ye've had enough for one day.'

'I haven't done anything for you.'

'Nor you have, kidda, but you've been a change. Three months if I'm still here?'

It was only the next week that Mickey ended up in the medical ward. He was grey and *in extremis*, but still joking. 'You still here?' he said, recognising me. 'Aah thowt you'd be back in kindergarten.' I wish someone would say that to me today. However, little Geordie miners do not die easily. He struggled on for a few weeks, wearing a sort of nightie as he hated anything tight, and at night he also wore a bed cap – Sister christened him 'Wee Willy Winky.' He needed virtually continuous oxygen provided by an array of heavy black cylinders that surrounded his bed – he said that it felt like being in a U-boat. At night you could spot Mickey's cot by the bright glow of his woodbine, burning beautifully in almost pure oxygen. No one stopped him – they had grown to love him too much, and besides all the nurses smoked in those days, and I did, too. In fact a communal name for nurses on night duty was a fug. Mickey's spirit remained uncrushed by illness, and the haunted look of the dying was conspicuously absent – there was no reproach in his eyes. The only time I saw fear was shortly before he died. I was hurrying through my examination that day and he spotted it. 'Where's the fire, doc?' I told him it was my job to vaccinate all the hospital staff against flu that day and that I was already late. 'Well, aam dyin' and there is nowt to do but keep me comfy, so gan on and keep the livin' healthy, aam a bit fed up mind you, so if aam still around toneet promise you'll give me one them jabs you're givin.' It seemed an odd logic, but who was I to argue? I was about to go when he caught my hand and held it. 'Promise me, doc.' There was a brief glimpse of real fear deep in those black eyes, 'You won't let them bury me, will you? I will make a good blaze, but I couldn't stand all that earth on me for eternity – aave been under the ground too lang already. The missus wants me next to her lot on Hetton Hill, but aah want me ashes on Roker Park. Promise me.' So I did.

We were too efficient at immunising, as it turned out. We vaccinated all the staff in one frenetic day. It was the next day, when 50% of the nurses and doctors did not turn up for work because of reactions to the jab, that caused the crisis. Mickey joked that as there was no one to look after him it was time he went. He insisted on the flu jab and held my hand. 'A promise is a promise.' I nodded. He relaxed and died peacefully that night. His wife in fact told me that she would never bury him, as she understood his fear, and she promised to get one of their sons to take his ashes to the football ground. They did win the next home game. I have never had a flu jab since, but I often think of Mickey.